Obesity - Current Science and Clinical Approaches

Edited by Gitanjali Srivastava

Published in London, United Kingdom

Obesity - Current Science and Clinical Approaches
http://dx.doi.org/10.5772/intechopen.1006400
Edited by Gitanjali Srivastava

Contributors
Adriano Verame, Antonio Roberto Doro, Ashutosh Prasad Tripathi, Aylton Figueira Jr, Brijesh Kumar Singh, Carlos Eduardo Rosa da Silva, Diego Santiago, Eduardo Barbosa, Erildo Vicente Muller, Geetanjali Sethy, Gustavo Almeida, Hasan Ali, Leonardo Lima, Liz Elaine Sowek, Madhulika Tripathi, Mamata Panda, Manish Kumar Verma, Marcia Regina Carletto, Michele Mae Ann Yuen, Mohamad Hamoud, Punyatoya Samal, Wilian Santana

First published in London, United Kingdom, 2025 by IntechOpen
IntechOpen is the global imprint of INTECHOPEN LIMITED, registered in England and Wales, registration number: 11086078, 167-169 Great Portland Street, London, W1W 5PF, United Kingdom

For EU product safety concerns: IN TECH d.o.o., Prolaz Marije Krucifikse Kozulić 3, 51000 Rijeka, Croatia, info@intechopen.com or visit our website at intechopen.com.

British Library Cataloguing-in-Publication Data
A catalogue record for this book is available from the British Library

Obesity - Current Science and Clinical Approaches
Edited by Gitanjali Srivastava
p. cm.
Print ISBN 978-1-83635-112-2
Online ISBN 978-1-83635-111-5
eBook (PDF) ISBN 978-1-83635-113-9

If disposing of this product, please recycle the paper responsibly.

Meet the editor

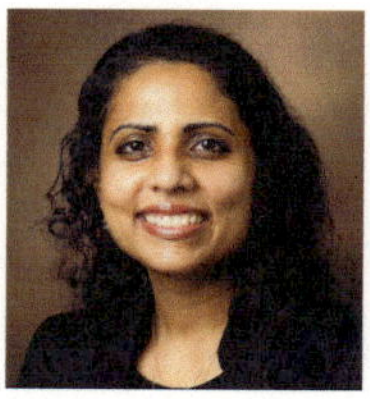

Gitanjali Srivastava, MD, is a Professor of Medicine, Pediatrics, and Surgery at Vanderbilt University School of Medicine. She serves as the Medical Director/Chief of Obesity Medicine, Program Director of the Obesity Medicine Fellowship, and Co-Director of the Vanderbilt Weight Loss Program. Dr. Srivastava is a Diplomate of the American Board of Obesity Medicine, Internal Medicine, and Pediatrics. She is Vice-Chair of the Obesity Medicine Fellowship Council and Tennessee's Expert for the Chronic Weight Management Task Force. An internationally recognized educator, researcher, and world-renowned adult and pediatric obesity medicine physician-scientist, Dr. Srivastava specializes in anti-obesity pharmacotherapy. She has authored numerous publications and developed models and curricula for obesity care. She earned her medical degree at LSU and completed fellowship training at Harvard Medical School.

Contents

Preface

Obesity is a complex and multifaceted condition that affects millions of individuals worldwide, transcending age, gender, and socioeconomic status. The chapters in this book aim to provide a comprehensive understanding of obesity, its complications, and the various approaches to its treatment and management, with a focus on integrative, multidisciplinary non-pharmacological strategies for obesity care. By exploring the latest research and clinical practices, we aim to provide valuable insights and practical strategies for healthcare professionals, researchers, and individuals interested in addressing this global health challenge.

Section 1: Understanding Obesity sets the foundation by delving into the causes, prevalence, and health complications associated with obesity. This section provides a comprehensive overview, helping readers understand the significant impact of obesity on overall health. It also addresses the unique challenges faced by children and adolescents, examining the psychological effects of obesity in these age groups and underscoring the importance of early intervention and mental health support.

Section 2: New Perspectives in Obesity Management and Treatment presents innovative approaches to treating obesity. From interdisciplinary proposals within the unified health system to aerobic and strength training strategies, this section highlights the collaborative efforts and technical advancements in obesity treatment. It also examines the role of mitochondrial health and the clinical applications of therapeutic fasting and natural supplements as innovative methods for enhancing health in obese individuals.

Section 3: Advanced Therapeutic Approaches for Obesity Care delves into cutting-edge treatments and interventions. This section covers topics such as the One-Anastomosis Gastric Bypass procedure and body contouring techniques like VASER liposuction, providing readers with a glimpse into the future of obesity management. It highlights the benefits and considerations of these advanced treatments, emphasizing the importance of holistic and integrative approaches to care.

Together, these chapters provide a comprehensive view of obesity, integrating theoretical knowledge with practical applications. We hope this book serves as a valuable resource for those dedicated to understanding and addressing obesity, ultimately contributing to better health and well-being for individuals affected by this condition.

Gitanjali Srivastava, MD, FACP, FAAP, FTOS, DABOM
Professor of Medicine, Pediatrics and Surgery,
Division of Diabetes, Endocrinology and Metabolism,
Department of Medicine,
Vanderbilt University School of Medicine,
Nashville, TN, USA

Section 1

Understanding Obesity

Chapter 1

Obesity and Its Complications

Michele Mae Ann Yuen

Abstract

Obesity is associated with many health complications, which are attributable to several mechanistic changes that take place as excess adipose tissue builds up in the body. These changes include chronic inflammation, oxidative stress, insulin resistance, endothelial dysfunction, elevated levels of growth-promoting adipokines, mechanical effects of excess adiposity due to ectopic deposition and direct loading, and heightened activities of the renin-angiotensin-aldosterone system (RAAS) and sympathetic nervous system (SNS). These mechanistic processes may occur in isolation or in combination to contribute to the development of obesity-associated comorbidities. Understanding the full spectrum of obesity-associated comorbidities will help to guide the clinical assessment as well as treatment and monitoring of individuals with obesity. This chapter will include a review of the current evidence in relation to the scope of obesity-associated comorbidities and discussions on how excess adiposity can contribute to their pathogenesis.

Keywords: obesity-associated comorbidities, mechanistic changes, inflammation, oxidative stress, insulin resistance, mechanical effects, RAAS and SNS activations, literature review

1. Introduction

Obesity is a chronic disease characterized by excessive adiposity, with or without abnormal distribution or function of the adipose tissue [1]. Accumulation of adipose tissues has been associated with numerous complications that transverse multiple organ systems and specialties in clinical medicine [2]. The pathophysiological linkages between excessive adiposity and its complications have not been completely elucidated, but evidence so far has supported several possible mechanisms, including chronic inflammation and oxidative stress (in association with insulin resistance, endothelial dysfunction, and growth promotion by adipokines), mechanical effects due to ectopic fat infiltration and direct loading effect of excessive adiposity, and activation of the renin-angiotensin-aldosterone system and the sympathetic nervous system [2].

Expansion of adipose tissue can occur through hyperplasia (proliferation and differentiation of adipose precursor cells) or hypertrophy (increase in adipocyte size), with the proportion of each varying based on genetics, age, and environmental factors [3]. Different modes of fat accumulation have differential health effects, with the general presumption that adipocyte hypertrophy is more harmful than hyperplasia in the human body [3]. Adipose tissues can also be classified into "brown adipose tissue"

IntechOpen

(BAT) and "white adipose tissue" (WAT). BAT, characterized by the presence of uncoupling protein 1 (UCP1), is more abundant in infants compared to adults, and is involved in thermogenesis. BAT progressively becomes WAT with age. As WAT has greater capacity to expand by hypertrophy than BAT, which has limited lipid storage and undergoes apoptosis with expansion, the presence of WAT is associated with the adverse effects of obesity [4, 5]. Better understanding of the behavior of adipocytes and their interaction with the body will help to clarify and relate obesity to human health, especially in the context of the development of obesity complications. This chapter will review the linkage between obesity and its complications from a mechanistic point of view.

2. Chronic inflammation and oxidative stress in obesity

We now recognize that adipose tissue is not merely a storage site for excessive triglyceride but is a complex tissue containing a mixture of cell types (including fat cells, immune cells, endothelium, fibroblasts, neurons, and stem cells) that interact with one another [4]. Research in recent decades has identified adipose tissues as an endocrine organ that secretes various adipokines, including leptin, interleukin-6 (IL-6), tumor necrosis factor-α (TNF-α), monocyte chemoattractant protein-1 (MCP-1), resistin, and adiponectin, among others [4]. These adipokines primarily function to inform the body of its energy and nutritional status, thereby allowing for a coordinated control of food intake, energy expenditure, and metabolism [6]. In a dysregulated state such as obesity, these adipokines, in both independent and interactive manners, induce chronic low-grade inflammation. While inflammation in a controlled fashion is beneficial and functions to contain and eradicate threats to the host organism, chronic inflammation threatens health and is one possible mechanism by which obesity complications develop.

Leptin was the first adipokine to be discovered in 1994 as a product of the ob gene [7]. Secreted predominantly from adipose tissue, leptin serves to inform the brain of the presence of nutrition and promotes fed-state metabolic responses. Leptin deficiency in ob/ob mice and in humans with monogenic mutation leads to severe obesity; however, in the majority of cases, human obesity is marked by leptin resistance with elevated circulating levels of leptin [8, 9]. Leptin is a pro-inflammatory molecule, modulating both innate and adaptive immune responses, and is possibly one of the many links between obesity and chronic low-grade inflammation [10].

Interleukin-6 involvement in the inflammatory process is less clear-cut. Nonetheless, it had been demonstrated that muscle-derived IL-6 exhibits anti-inflammatory effects, whereas IL-6 produced by adipocytes promotes inflammation, and the expression of adipocyte-derived IL-6 and its receptor is elevated in obesity [11, 12]. The increased expression of adipocyte-derived IL-6 and its receptor in obesity is correlated with markers of macrophage infiltration and low-grade inflammation [12, 13]. IL-6 also stimulates the production of C-reactive protein (CRP) in human liver cells, potentially serving as a mediator or marker of inflammatory processes in the disease state [14, 15].

TNF-α promotes inflammation, and higher expressions of its messenger RNA (mRNA) have been detected in fat biopsy samples from individuals with obesity [16]. MCP-1, produced mainly in adipocytes, is a potent chemotactic factor for monocytes and activator of T helper cells, and its expression is increased in adipose tissue in individuals with obesity [17, 18]. Additionally, omental fat layer in individuals with severe obesity was found to have higher MCP-1 expression compared with subcutaneous fat layers, suggestive of a role of central obesity in promoting inflammation [18]. Resistin is primarily expressed in monocytic cells, rather than adipose tissue. Increased macrophage infiltration in adipose tissue in obesity is likely how resistin contributes to the chronic low-grade inflammation [19].

In contrast to the other adipokines, adiponectin has anti-inflammatory properties. However, its circulating levels are inversely related to mean adipocyte diameter, suggesting that adipocyte hypertrophy would impede the secretion of adiponectin [20]. Functional recovery of adiponectin secretion has been documented after about 10% weight loss in individuals with severe obesity (BMI $\geq$ 40 kg/m^2) [21].

Obesity induces oxidative stress by heightening the production of reactive oxygen species (ROS) in adipose tissue, increasing nicotinamide adenine dinucleotide phosphate (NADPH) oxidase expression and reducing levels of antioxidant enzymes [22]. Oxidative stress in obesity further contributes to the dysregulation of adipocytokines, including adiponectin, IL-6, and MCP-1 [22]. The synergistic effect of chronic inflammation and oxidative stress is implicated in metabolic disorders, as well as orthopedic, obstetric, dermatological, otorhinolaryngological, and even psychiatric comorbidities of obesity.

2.1 Obesity-associated chronic inflammation and oxidative stress and insulin resistance

Chronic inflammation and oxidative stress associated with obesity are implicated in insulin resistance, which in turn gives rise to multiple metabolic disorders, including type 2 diabetes, hypercholesterolemia, hypertriglyceridemia, and metabolic dysfunction-associated fatty liver disease (MAFLD) [23–25]. For instance, TNF-α interferes with normal insulin signaling by reducing tyrosine phosphorylation of insulin receptor in skeletal muscles and is implicated as a mediator of insulin resistance in obesity [26]. Resistin has been linked to insulin resistance and hypertension via activation of the Toll-like receptor 4 (TLR4)/P65/angiotensinogen (AGT) pathway and in turn, the renin-angiotensin system (RAS) in mice models [27]. In humans, resistin induces TNF-α and various interleukins, including interleukin 1β (IL-1β), IL-6, interleukin 8 (IL-8), and interleukin 12 (IL-12) that stimulate pro-inflammatory response [28]. Human resistin also induces the secretion of MCP-1 and activation of nuclear factor kappa B (NF-κB) to further promote inflammation [28].

In synergism with inflammation, reactive oxygen species (ROS) further aggravates insulin resistance in peripheral tissues by influencing insulin receptor signaling through multiple pathways. These changes cumulate in the decreased expression of glucose transporter type 4 (GLUT4) transporters, which are the primary glucose transporters in the cellular membranes of insulin-sensitive peripheral tissues, causing insulin resistance [29]. Insulin resistance, in turn, plays a role in the entire range of metabolic dysfunction-associated fatty liver diseases (MAFLD), from simple steatosis to metabolic dysfunction-associated steatohepatitis (MASH) and cirrhosis, which can potentially lead to liver cancer [30]. Insulin resistance in obesity is also implicated in dermatological conditions, such as acanthosis nigricans, acrochordons, and keratosis pilaris, and even frailty-related conditions in the elderly such as sarcopenia [31–33].

2.2 Endothelial dysfunction and obesity-associated chronic inflammation and oxidative stress

Endothelial dysfunction is another consequence of obesity-associated chronic inflammation and oxidative stress due to an increase in cell-surface adhesion molecules' expression and impairment in endothelium-dependent vascular relaxation [34]. Endothelial dysfunction represents a critical initiating factor in the development of atherosclerosis and associated cardiovascular pathologies, such as stable/unstable angina, acute myocardial infarction, coronary artery disease, and ischemic cerebrovascular events [35–38]. This pathological state further extends beyond cardiovascular diseases, contributing to hypertensive complications in pregnancy like gestational hypertension, preeclampsia, and eclampsia through impaired vascular regulation [39].

3. Adipokines and growth promotion

Some adipokines, such as insulin-like growth factor 1 (IGF-1) and leptin, have growth-promoting properties. In conjunction with sex-hormone alterations induced by excessive adiposity, obesity creates a pro-tumorigenic environment that has been implicated in the pathogenesis of over 20 distinct cancers. Colon cancer, for instance, is increased by 25–57% in overweight and obesity, and has been linked to elevation in IGF-1 and leptin and decreased adiponectin with increased adiposity [40–42]. Pancreatic cancer is increased up to 1.6 times in overweight and 3.5 times in obesity, with this association primarily driven by metabolic disturbances, such as systemic hyperinsulinemia and heightened insulin secretion from pancreatic β-cells [43–46]. These conditions activate insulin receptor signaling pathways in pancreatic acinar cells, promoting excessive digestive enzyme production, chronic inflammation, and subsequent transformation of precancerous lesion [47]. The sustained mitogenic effects of elevated insulin levels further accelerate the proliferation of neoplastic pancreatic cells [47].

Breast cancer risk is increased by 33% in postmenopausal women with obesity compared to those with normal body weight [48]. Adipose tissue takes over as the predominant site of estrogen production after menopause, and it follows that postmenopausal women with obesity have greater exposure to estrogen and its pro-tumorigenic effects [49]. Elevated leptin level is another mechanistic link between obesity and breast cancer. *In vitro* study found that stimulation of leptin receptors supported stem cell-like properties of breast cancer cells and preserved their self-renewal ability, thereby facilitating recurrence and metastasis [50].

Increased adiposity further contributes to the pool of bioactive estrogen in both women and men by increasing aromatase activity and reducing sex-hormone binding globulin (SHBG) [51]. Elevated estrogen level is linked to endometrial and epithelial ovarian cancer in women and prostate cancer in men [51–53]. In the context of elevation in leptin, obesity has been further linked to papillary, follicular, and anaplastic thyroid cancers via this mechanism [54, 55].

This discussion is by no means exhaustive of all the cancers that are linked to obesity. Other cancers that have been observed to occur at a higher incidence in obesity, from head to toe, include meningioma, glioma, esophageal adenocarcinoma and squamous cell carcinoma, gastric cardia high-grade dysplasia and adenocarcinoma, appendix carcinoid tumor, cholangiocarcinoma, extrahepatic bile duct cancer, gallbladder cancer, peritoneal cancer, renal cell carcinoma and transitional cell carcinoma, urothelial cell carcinoma and cutaneous melanoma [56–67]. The pathogenesis for some of these cancers in obesity is still not fully understood, but the pathological processes discussed in this and the following sections may have a contributory role to the development of some of these cancers.

4. Mechanical effects of increased adiposity

The mechanical effects of obesity refer to the ectopic distribution of fat with resulting end-organ damage and dysfunction and the direct effect of excess adiposity. Both mechanisms and the resulting complications will be discussed.

4.1 Ectopic fat deposition with organ injury and functional impairment

Excess fat in obesity may be deposited ectopically in organs, such as the liver, kidneys, pancreas, and heart. Within the liver, ectopic fat accumulation leads to metabolic dysfunction-associated fatty liver disease (MAFLD), a condition that can progress to nonalcoholic steatohepatitis (NASH), cirrhosis, and potentially hepatocellular carcinoma (HCC) [30, 68]. In the kidneys, ectopic fat deposition contributes to the development of "fatty kidney," increasing the risk of albuminuria or proteinuria, glomerulonephritis, chronic kidney disease, and end-stage renal failure [69]. Peri- and intra-pancreatic fat deposition is hypothesized to play a role in the pathogenesis of acute pancreatitis in individuals with obesity, though heightened lipolysis due to insulin resistance and chronic low-grade inflammation may also exacerbate this process [70, 71]. Cardiac ectopic fat deposition is associated with structural changes such as left atrial enlargement, which elevates the risk of atrial fibrillation, while excessive epicardial adipose tissue impairs ventricular contractility and may significantly contribute to nonischemic heart failure in overweight and obese individuals [72–74]. Beyond these organ-specific effects, ectopic fat deposition is linked to broader obesity-associated comorbidities, including carpal tunnel syndrome (possibly due to compression of the median nerve by excess adipose tissue) and osteoporosis (possibly due to fat infiltration of the bone marrow secondary to unbalanced differentiation of the common progenitor towards adipocytes rather than osteoblasts) [75, 76].

4.2 Excess adiposity and direct loading effect

Physical effect of excess adiposity can also affect bodily functions directly. For example, fat buildup in the neck area narrows the upper airways and makes the pharynx more prone to collapsing, while central obesity decreases lung capacity and reduces the downward pull on the upper airway [77]. These anatomical changes increase the risk of developing obstructive sleep apnea (OSA) [77]. Excess fat in the abdominal area is linked to more frequent relaxations of the lower esophageal sphincter, disruptions in the pressure at the esophagogastric junction, and a higher gastroesophageal pressure gradient, all of which contribute to gastroesophageal reflux disease (GERD) and its complications like erosive esophagitis and Barrett's esophagus [78]. Consequently, esophageal and gastric adenocarcinomas, partly caused by GERD, are also more common in individuals with obesity [79, 80]. Additionally, increased fat around the chest and chronic inflammation, along with other factors such as GERD, play a role in obesity-related asthma [81].

Excessive body fat impacts joint loading patterns, which in turn can trigger inflammation in cartilage and bones and increase the risk of osteoarthritis (OA) in both weight-bearing joints (such as knees and hips) and non-weight-bearing joints (like the hands) [82]. Additionally, individuals with obesity may experience a shift in their center of gravity, making them more prone to injuries and fractures, particularly in the clavicle, upper limbs, hips, and lower limbs [83, 84].

Obesity also exerts mechanical impact that contributes to several skin-related issues. For example, enlarged skinfolds create localized occlusion, trapping heat and moisture, which, combined with friction between skin surfaces, heightens the likelihood of conditions like intertrigo and hidradenitis suppurativa [31]. The added weight on the lower limbs raises the risk of stasis-related skin problems, such as cellulitis, lymphedema, and elephantiasis nostras verrucosa [85, 86]. Similarly, the pressure on the soles can lead to plantar hyperkeratosis [31]. Additionally, the stretching of the skin due to obesity increases the chances of developing striae distensae [31].

Excessive adiposity can directly contribute to neurogenic pain disorders, including ulnar nerve compression and meralgia paresthetica [87, 88]. Meralgia paresthetica specifically results from the compression of the lateral femoral cutaneous nerve due to abnormal accumulation of abdominal fat [88]. Elevated intra-abdominal pressure is additionally linked to several urological issues, such as nocturia, overactive bladder, and both stress and urge urinary incontinence in women [89–92].

Other obesity-related health complications resulting from mechanical effects of adipose tissue include chronic leg pain, intervertebral disc disorder with lower back pain, atelectasis, hiatal and ventral hernia, pressure ulcer, fecal incontinence in female, and venous insufficiency [2].

5. Increased activation of renin-angiotensin-aldosterone system (RAAS) and sympathetic nervous system (SNS)

Both the renin-angiotensin-aldosterone system (RAAS) and the sympathetic nervous system (SNS) seem to be in overdrive in obesity, potentially contributing to the onset of hypertension [93, 94]. Additionally, changes in fluid and sodium balance that favor higher blood pressure in obesity may further exacerbate this condition [95]. Hypertension and other hemodynamic alterations promote the development of left ventricular hypertrophy in obesity [96]. These factors, combined with atherosclerosis, could explain the heightened risk of sudden cardiac death in individuals with obesity [97]. Moreover, excessive sweating (hyperhidrosis) in obesity has been linked to elevated RAAS and SNS activity [98]. Lastly, RAAS activation might play a role in some symptoms of premenstrual syndrome, which is more common in those with obesity [99].

6. Others and unknown

Obesity also weakens immunity, alters brain structure, raises cortisol levels, and increases uric acid [100, 101]. These changes result in higher infection risks, manic episodes in bipolar disorder, depression, and gout in obesity, respectively. Connections are also observed between obesity and anxiety and panic disorders, headache disorders, thiamine deficiency, and additional pregnancy-related issues, such as cervical incompetence and polyhydramnios, among others [100, 101]. The exact ways in which obesity contributes to these conditions are not yet fully

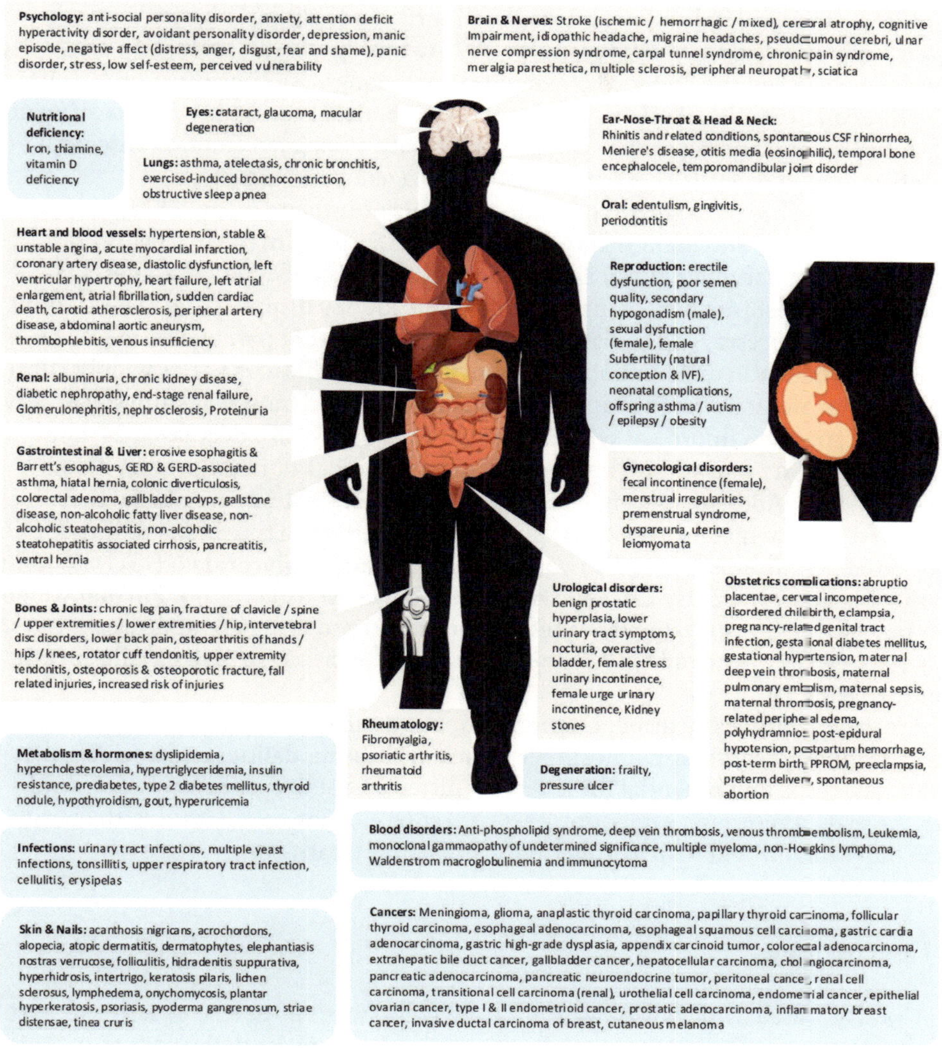

Figure 1.
Summary of obesity-associated comorbidities (adapted from Ref. [2]).

understood. Although proving a direct cause-and-effect relationship between excess body fat and these disorders is challenging, the fact that many improve or resolve with weight loss suggests that obesity plays a significant role.

The currently identified health complications associated with obesity are summarized in **Figure 1**. It should be recognized that the entirety of the health impact of obesity is much more complex than depicted in this chapter. As more evidence emerge, our understanding of the full effect of obesity on health will continue to evolve.

7. Evaluating and treating obesity and its complications

The harm that excessive adiposity poses to the human body is well recognized but the criteria for diagnosis and identifying individuals for treatment remain controversial. The limitations of using body mass index as a measure for obesity have long been discussed. A revised definition and diagnostic criteria of clinical obesity were proposed and published in *Lancet* in January 2025 to incorporate an evaluation of obesity symptoms, defined the presence of complications along with consideration of the structural and functional effects they have on the body, in recommending treatment [1]. A full understanding of the spectrum of obesity-associated comorbidities will be beneficial, if not eventually essential, in the management of obesity.

Weight loss has been shown to reduce markers of inflammation, oxidative stress, insulin resistance, and endothelial dysfunction [102–104]. In the real-world setting, weight reduction has been shown to reduce the risk of type 2 diabetes, OSA, hypertension dyslipidemia, asthma, and chronic kidney disease [105]. The amount of weight loss necessary to bring about reversal of different pathogenic mechanisms and improvement in different obesity-associated comorbidities varies widely [106]. Magkos et al. demonstrated that adipose tissue, liver, and muscle insulin sensitivity, and β-cell function improved with 5% weight loss, which also decreased 24-hour ambulatory heart rate and 24-hour ambulatory systolic, but not diastolic, blood pressure [107]. Additional weight loss up to 16% of initial body weight further improved muscle insulin sensitivity and reduced fat-free mass, fat mass, intra-abdominal adipose tissue (IAAT) volume, intrahepatic triglyceride (IHTG) content, fasting plasma insulin, leptin, and triglyceride concentrations [107]. Further weight loss beyond 16% of initial body weight was necessary to bring about decrease in plasma-free fatty acid and CRP concentrations and increase in plasma adiponectin concentration [107].

Treatment of obesity through weight reduction can be achieved through diet, exercise, pharmacotherapy, and surgery. Each of these modalities carries different efficacies, risks, and potential for reversing different obesity-associated comorbidities. As such, a thorough evaluation of health complications associated with obesity in each individual would help to guide and personalize treatment.

8. Conclusions

Obesity is associated with over 200 health complications that span across almost all organ systems. The pathogenesis of these complications is attributable to various mechanistic changes that are seen with the accumulation of excessive adiposity in the human body. These mechanistic changes seem to be reversible with weight loss, with different magnitudes of weight loss necessary for different pathogenic processes. Reversal of obesity-associated comorbidities follows the correction of these mechanistic changes in weight loss. Having a better understanding of the obesity-associated comorbidities will be useful to guide clinical assessment and treatment of affected individuals.

Acknowledgements

Special acknowledgments to Joseph Brancale, Nitya Kadambi, and the Obesity Comorbidity Collaborative for their contributions to the generation of the list of obesity-associated comorbidities, and to Lee M. Kaplan for the conceptualization and supervision of this project. The contributors to this work were at the Obesity, Metabolism and Nutrition Institute, Department of Medicine, Massachusetts General Hospital during the initial phase of this project.

DOI: http://dx.doi.org/10.5772/intechopen.1010254

Conflict of interest

The author declares no conflict of interest.

Author details

Michele Mae Ann Yuen
The University of Hong Kong, Hong Kong SAR

*Address all correspondence to: micheleyuen@gmail.com

References

[1] Rubino F, Cummings DE, Eckel RH, Cohen RV, Wilding JPH, Brown WA, et al. Definition and diagnostic criteria of clinical obesity. The Lancet Diabetes and Endocrinology. 2025;**13**(3):221-262

[2] Yuen MMA. Health complications of obesity: 224 obesity-associated comorbidities from a mechanistic perspective. Gastroenterology Clinics of North America. 2023;**52**(2):363-380

[3] Horwitz A, Birk R. Adipose tissue hyperplasia and hypertrophy in common and syndromic obesity-the case of BBS obesity. Nutrients. 2023;**15**(15):3445

[4] Cohen P, Spiegelman BM. Cell biology of fat storage. Molecular Biology of the Cell. 2016;**27**(16):2523-2527

[5] Kotzbeck P, Giordano A, Mondini E, Murano I, Severi I, Venema W, et al. Brown adipose tissue whitening leads to brown adipocyte death and adipose tissue inflammation. Journal of Lipid Research. 2018;**59**(5):784-794

[6] Pereira SSA-L, Adipokines JI. Biological functions and metabolically healthy obese profile. Journal of Receptor Ligand and Channel Research. 2014;**7**:15-25

[7] Zhang Y, Proenca R, Maffei M, Barone M, Leopold L, Friedman JM. Positional cloning of the mouse obese gene and its human homologue. Nature. 1994;**372**(6505):425-432

[8] Montague CT, Farooqi IS, Whitehead JP, Soos MA, Rau H, Wareham NJ, et al. Congenital leptin deficiency is associated with severe early-onset obesity in humans. Nature. 1997;**387**(6636):903-908

[9] Perakakis N, Farr OM, Mantzoros CS. Leptin in leanness and obesity: JACC state-of-the-art review. Journal of the American College of Cardiology. 2021;**77**(6):745-760

[10] Abella V, Scotece M, Conde J, Pino J, Gonzalez-Gay MA, Gomez-Reino JJ, et al. Leptin in the interplay of inflammation, metabolism and immune system disorders. Nature Reviews Rheumatology. 2017;**13**(2):100-109

[11] Nara H, Watanabe R. Anti-inflammatory effect of muscle-derived Interleukin-6 and its involvement in lipid metabolism. International Journal of Molecular Sciences. 2021;**22**(18):9889

[12] Sindhu S, Thomas R, Shihab P, Sriraman D, Behbehani K, Ahmad R. Obesity is a positive modulator of IL-6R and IL-6 expression in the subcutaneous adipose tissue: Significance for metabolic inflammation. PLoS One. 2015;**10**(7):e0133494

[13] Weisberg SP, McCann D, Desai M, Rosenbaum M, Leibel RL, Ferrante AW Jr. Obesity is associated with macrophage accumulation in adipose tissue. The Journal of Clinical Investigation. 2003;**112**(12):1796-1808

[14] Castell JV, Gomez-Lechon MJ, David M, Hirano T, Kishimoto T, Heinrich PC. Recombinant human interleukin-6 (IL-6/BSF-2/HSF) regulates the synthesis of acute phase proteins in human hepatocytes. FEBS Letters. 1988;**232**(2):347-350

[15] Ansar W, Ghosh S. C-reactive protein and the biology of disease. Immunologic Research. 2013;**56**(1):131-142

[16] Kern PA, Saghizadeh M, Ong JM, Bosch RJ, Deem R, Simsolo RB. The

expression of tumor necrosis factor in human adipose tissue. Regulation by obesity, weight loss, and relationship to lipoprotein lipase. The Journal of Clinical Investigation. 1995;**95**(5):2111-2119

[17] Singh S, Anshita D, Ravichandiran V. MCP-1: Function, regulation, and involvement in disease. International Immunopharmacology. 2021;**101**(Pt B):107598

[18] Panee J. Monocyte chemoattractant protein 1 (MCP-1) in obesity and diabetes. Cytokine. 2012;**60**(1):1-12

[19] Al Hannan F, Culligan KG. Human resistin and the RELM of inflammation in diabesity. Diabetology and Metabolic Syndrome. 2015;7:54

[20] Drolet R, Belanger C, Fortier M, Huot C, Mailloux J, Legare D, et al. Fat depot-specific impact of visceral obesity on adipocyte adiponectin release in women. Obesity (Silver Spring). 2009;**17**(3):424-430

[21] De Rosa A, Monaco ML, Capasso M, Forestieri P, Pilone V, Nardelli C, et al. Adiponectin oligomers as potential indicators of adipose tissue improvement in obese subjects. European Journal of Endocrinology. 2013;**169**(1):37-43

[22] Furukawa S, Fujita T, Shimabukuro M, Iwaki M, Yamada Y, Nakajima Y, et al. Increased oxidative stress in obesity and its impact on metabolic syndrome. The Journal of Clinical Investigation. 2004;**114**(12):1752-1761

[23] Kahn SE, Hull RL, Utzschneider KM. Mechanisms linking obesity to insulin resistance and type 2 diabetes. Nature. 2006;**444**(7121):840-846

[24] Klop B, Elte JW, Cabezas MC. Dyslipidemia in obesity: Mechanisms and potential targets. Nutrients. 2013;**5**(4):1218-1240

[25] Stefan N, Yki-Jarvinen H, Neuschwander-Tetri BA. Metabolic dysfunction-associated steatotic liver disease: Heterogeneous pathomechanisms and effectiveness of metabolism-based treatment. The Lancet Diabetes and Endocrinology. 2025;**13**(2):134-148

[26] Cheung AT, Ree D, Kolls JK, Fuselier J, Coy DH, Bryer-Ash M. An in vivo model for elucidation of the mechanism of tumor necrosis factor-alpha (TNF-alpha)-induced insulin resistance: Evidence for differential regulation of insulin signaling by TNF-alpha. Endocrinology. 1998;**139**(12):4928-4935

[27] Jiang Y, Lu L, Hu Y, Li Q, An C, Yu X, et al. Resistin induces hypertension and insulin resistance in mice via a TLR4-dependent pathway. Scientific Reports. 2016;**6**:22193

[28] Tripathi D, Kant S, Pandey S, Ehtesham NZ. Resistin in metabolism, inflammation, and disease. The FEBS Journal. 2020;**287**(15):3141-3149

[29] Hurrle S, Hsu WH. The etiology of oxidative stress in insulin resistance. Biomed Journal. 2017;**40**(5):257-262

[30] Loomba R, Friedman SL, Shulman GI. Mechanisms and disease consequences of nonalcoholic fatty liver disease. Cell. 2021;**184**(10):2537-2564

[31] Darlenski R, Mihaylova V, Handjieva-Darlenska T. The link between obesity and the skin. Frontiers in Nutrition. 2022;**9**:855573

[32] Shah R, Jindal A, Patel N. Acrochordons as a cutaneous sign of metabolic syndrome: A case-control

study. Annals of Medical and Health Sciences Research. 2014;**4**(2):202-205

[33] Cleasby ME, Jamieson PM, Atherton PJ. Insulin resistance and sarcopenia: Mechanistic links between common co-morbidities. The Journal of Endocrinology. 2016;**229**(2):R67-R81

[34] Stenvinkel P. Endothelial dysfunction and inflammation—Is there a link? Nephrology, Dialysis, Transplantation. 2001;**16**(10):1968-1971

[35] Powell-Wiley TM, Poirier P, Burke LE, Despres JP, Gordon-Larsen P, Lavie CJ, et al. Obesity and cardiovascular disease: A scientific statement from the American Heart Association. Circulation. 2021;**143**(21):e984-e1010

[36] Rajendran K, Devarajan N, Ganesan M, Ragunathan M. Obesity, inflammation and acute myocardial infarction - expression of leptin, IL-6 and high sensitivity-CRP in Chennai based population. Thrombosis Journal. 2012;**10**(1):13

[37] Van Gaal LF, Mertens IL, De Block CE. Mechanisms linking obesity with cardiovascular disease. Nature. 2006;**444**(7121):875-880

[38] Kernan WN, Inzucchi SE, Sawan C, Macko RF, Furie KL. Obesity: A stubbornly obvious target for stroke prevention. Stroke. 2013;**44**(1):278-286

[39] Spradley FT, Palei AC, Granger JP. Increased risk for the development of preeclampsia in obese pregnancies: Weighing in on the mechanisms. American Journal of Physiology. Regulatory, Integrative and Comparative Physiology. 2015;**309**(11):R1326-R1343

[40] Ungvari Z, Fekete M, Varga P, Lehoczki A, Fekete JT, Ungvari A, et al. Overweight and obesity significantly increase colorectal cancer risk: A meta-analysis of 66 studies revealing a 25-57% elevation in risk. Geroscience. 2024

[41] Lahm H, Suardet L, Laurent PL, Fischer JR, Ceyhan A, Givel JC, et al. Growth regulation and co-stimulation of human colorectal cancer cell lines by insulin-like growth factor I, II and transforming growth factor alpha. British Journal of Cancer. 1992;**65**(3):341-346

[42] Ye P, Xi Y, Huang Z, Xu P. Linking obesity with colorectal cancer: Epidemiology and mechanistic insights. Cancers (Basel). 2020;**12**(6)

[43] Stolzenberg-Solomon RZ, Schairer C, Moore S, Hollenbeck A, Silverman DT. Lifetime adiposity and risk of pancreatic cancer in the NIH-AARP diet and health study cohort. The American Journal of Clinical Nutrition. 2013;**98**(4):1057-1065

[44] Fryzek JP, Schenk M, Kinnard M, Greenson JK, Garabrant DH. The association of body mass index and pancreatic cancer in residents of southeastern Michigan, 1996-1999. American Journal of Epidemiology. 2005;**162**(3):222-228

[45] Berrington de Gonzalez A, Sweetland S, Spencer E. A meta-analysis of obesity and the risk of pancreatic cancer. British Journal of Cancer. 2003;**89**(3):519-523

[46] Lin Y, Kikuchi S, Tamakoshi A, Yagyu K, Obata Y, Inaba Y, et al. Obesity, physical activity and the risk of pancreatic cancer in a large Japanese cohort. International Journal of Cancer. 2007;**120**(12):2665-2671

[47] Eibl G, Rozengurt E. Obesity and pancreatic cancer: Insight into mechanisms. Cancers (Basel). 2021;**13**(20):5067

[48] Chen Y, Liu L, Zhou Q, Imam MU, Cai J, Wang Y, et al. Body mass index had different effects on premenopausal and postmenopausal breast cancer risks: A dose-response meta-analysis with 3,318,796 subjects from 31 cohort studies. BMC Public Health. 2017;**17**(1):936

[49] Devericks EN, Carson MS, McCullough LE, Coleman MF, Hursting SD. The obesity-breast cancer link: A multidisciplinary perspective. Cancer Metastasis Reviews. 2022;**41**(3):607-625

[50] Zheng Q, Banaszak L, Fracci S, Basali D, Dunlap SM, Hursting SD, et al. Leptin receptor maintains cancer stem-like properties in triple negative breast cancer cells. Endocrine-Related Cancer. 2013;**20**(6):797-808

[51] Onstad MA, Schmandt RE, Lu KH. Addressing the role of obesity in endometrial cancer risk, prevention, and treatment. Journal of Clinical Oncology. 2016;**34**(35):4225-4230

[52] Dai L, Song K, Di W. Adipocytes: Active facilitators in epithelial ovarian cancer progression? Journal of Ovarian Research. 2020;**13**(1):115

[53] Parikesit D, Mochtar CA, Umbas R, Hamid AR. The impact of obesity towards prostate diseases. Prostate International. 2016;**4**(1):1-6

[54] Kim WG, Cheng SY. Mechanisms linking obesity and thyroid cancer development and progression in mouse models. Hormones and Cancer. 2018;**9**(2):108-116

[55] Masone S, Velotti N, Savastano S, Filice E, Serao R, Vitiello A, et al. Morbid obesity and thyroid cancer rate. A review of literature. Journal of Clinical Medicine. 2021;**10**(9):1894

[56] Khazanchi R, Nandoliya KR, Shahin MN, Rae AI, Chaliparambil RK, Bowden SG, et al. Obesity and meningioma: A US population-based study paired with analysis of a multi-institutional cohort. Journal of Neurosurgery. 2024;**140**(6):1558-1567

[57] Ahn S, Han K, Lee JE, Jeun SS, Park YM, Yang SH. Associations of general and abdominal obesity with the risk of glioma development. Cancers (Basel). 2021;**13**(12):2859

[58] Lindkvist B, Johansen D, Stocks T, Concin H, Bjorge T, Almquist M, et al. Metabolic risk factors for esophageal squamous cell carcinoma and adenocarcinoma: A prospective study of 580,000 subjects within the me-can project. BMC Cancer. 2014;**14**:103

[59] Huang YK, Kang WM, Ma ZQ, Liu YQ, Zhou L, Yu JC. Body mass index, serum total cholesterol, and risk of gastric high-grade dysplasia: A case-control study among Chinese adults. Medicine (Baltimore). 2016;**95**(35):e4730

[60] Kim HJ, Kim N, Kim HY, Lee HS, Yoon H, Shin CM, et al. Relationship between body mass index and the risk of early gastric cancer and dysplasia regardless of helicobacter pylori infection. Gastric Cancer. 2015;**18**(4):762-773

[61] Lan X, Fazio N, Abdel-Rahman O. Exploring the relationship between obesity, metabolic syndrome and neuroendocrine neoplasms. Metabolites. 2022;**12**(11):1150

[62] Parsi MA. Obesity and cholangiocarcinoma. World Journal of Gastroenterology. 2013;**19**(4):457-462

[63] Saeed U, Nordsletten M, Myklebust TA, Robsahm TE, Moller B, Skalhegg BS, et al. Cancer risk and survival

according to body mass index in hepatobiliary malignancies: A nationwide registry-based cohort study. Hepato-Pancreato-Biliary. 2023;**25**(11):1382-1392

[64] van de Vlasakker VCJ, van Erning FN, Lurvink RJ, de Hingh I, Nienhuijs SW. The impact of body weight on the development of peritoneal metastases in colorectal cancer patients: Results from a nationwide cohort study. World Journal of Surgical Oncology. 2023;**21**(1):328

[65] Chow WH, Gridley G, Fraumeni JF Jr, Jarvholm B. Obesity, hypertension, and the risk of kidney cancer in men. The New England Journal of Medicine. 2000;**343**(18):1305-1311

[66] Papavasileiou G, Tsilingiris D, Spyrou N, Vallianou NG, Karampela I, Magkos F, et al. Obesity and main urologic cancers: Current systematic evidence, novel biological mechanisms, perspectives and challenges. Seminars in Cancer Biology. 2023;**91**:70-98

[67] Almeida, Oliveira F, Klose J, Schulze HJ, Ribeiro Teixeira M, Dermietzel A, Wellenbrock S, et al. The influence of obesity on melanoma and sentinel lymph node diagnosis: A retrospective monocentric study in 1001 patients. Cancers (Basel). 2023;**15**(6):1806

[68] Rajesh Y, Sarkar D. Molecular mechanisms regulating obesity-associated hepatocellular carcinoma. Cancers (Basel). 2020;**12**(5):1290

[69] Kambham N, Markowitz GS, Valeri AM, Lin J, D'Agati VD. Obesity-related glomerulopathy: An emerging epidemic. Kidney International. 2001;**59**(4):1498-1509

[70] Wiese ML, Aghdassi AA, Lerch MM, Steveling A. Excess body weight and pancreatic disease. Visceral Medicine. 2021;**37**(4):281-286

[71] Cho SK, Huh JH, Yoo JS, Kim JW, Lee KJ. HOMA-estimated insulin resistance as an independent prognostic factor in patients with acute pancreatitis. Scientific Reports. 2019;**9**(1):14894

[72] Lavie CJ, Pandey A, Lau DH, Alpert MA, Sanders P. Obesity and atrial fibrillation prevalence, pathogenesis, and prognosis: Effects of weight loss and exercise. Journal of the American College of Cardiology. 2017;**70**(16):2022-2035

[73] Rayner JJ, Banerjee R, Holloway CJ, Lewis AJM, Peterzan MA, Francis JM, et al. The relative contribution of metabolic and structural abnormalities to diastolic dysfunction in obesity. International Journal of Obesity. 2018;**42**(3):441-447

[74] Ebong IA, Goff DC Jr, Rodriguez CJ, Chen H, Bertoni AG. Mechanisms of heart failure in obesity. Obesity Research & Clinical Practice. 2014;**8**(6):e540-e548

[75] Lampainen K, Shiri R, Auvinen J, Karppinen J, Ryhanen J, Hulkkonen S. Weight-related and personal risk factors of carpal tunnel syndrome in the northern Finland birth cohort 1966. Journal of Clinical Medicine. 2022;**11**(6):1510

[76] Gkastaris K, Goulis DG, Potoupnis M, Anastasilakis AD, Kapetanos G. Obesity, osteoporosis and bone metabolism. Journal of Musculoskeletal & Neuronal Interactions. 2020;**20**(3):372-381

[77] Schwartz AR, Patil SP, Laffan AM, Polotsky V, Schneider H, Smith PL. Obesity and obstructive sleep apnea: Pathogenic mechanisms and therapeutic approaches. Proceedings of the American Thoracic Society. 2008;**5**(2):185-192

[78] Wu JC, Mui LM, Cheung CM, Chan Y, Sung JJ. Obesity is associated with increased transient lower esophageal sphincter relaxation. Gastroenterology. 2007;**132**(3):883-889

[79] Alexandre L, Long E, Beales IL. Pathophysiological mechanisms linking obesity and esophageal adenocarcinoma. World Journal of Gastrointestinal Pathophysiology. 2014;**5**(4):534-549

[80] Karczewski J, Begier-Krasinska B, Staszewski R, Poplawska E, Gulczynska-Elhadi K, Dobrowolska A. Obesity and the risk of gastrointestinal cancers. Digestive Diseases and Sciences. 2019;**64**(10):2740-2749

[81] Baffi CW, Winnica DE, Holguin F. Asthma and obesity: Mechanisms and clinical implications. Asthma Research and Practice. 2015;**1**:1

[82] Reyes C, Leyland KM, Peat G, Cooper C, Arden NK, Prieto-Alhambra D. Association between overweight and obesity and risk of clinically diagnosed knee, hip, and hand osteoarthritis: A population-based cohort study. Arthritis & Rhematology. 2016;**68**(8):1869-1875

[83] Corbeil P, Simoneau M, Rancourt D, Tremblay A, Teasdale N. Increased risk for falling associated with obesity: Mathematical modeling of postural control. IEEE Transactions on Neural Systems and Rehabilitation Engineering. 2001;**9**(2):126-136

[84] Rinonapoli G, Pace V, Ruggiero C, Ceccarini P, Bisaccia M, Meccariello L, et al. Obesity and bone: A complex relationship. International Journal of Molecular Sciences. 2021;**22**(24):13662

[85] Cranendonk DR, Lavrijsen APM, Prins JM, Wiersinga WJ. Cellulitis: Current insights into pathophysiology and clinical management. The Netherlands Journal of Medicine. 2017;**75**(9):366-378

[86] Damstra RJ, Dickinson-Blok JL, Voesten HG. Shaving technique and compression therapy for elephantiasis Nostras Verrucosa (Lymphostatic Verrucosis) of forefeet and toes in end-stage primary lymphedema: A 5 year follow-up study in 28 patients and a review of the literature. Journal of Clinical Medicine. 2020;**9**(10):3139

[87] Descatha A, Leclerc A, Chastang JF, Roquelaure Y, Study Group on Repetitive W. Incidence of ulnar nerve entrapment at the elbow in repetitive work. Scandinavian Journal of Work, Environment & Health. 2004;**30**(3):234-240

[88] Deal CL, Canoso JJ. Meralgia paresthetica and large abdomens. Annals of Internal Medicine. 1982;**96**(6 Pt 1):787-788

[89] Moon S, Chung HS, Yu JM, Ko KJ, Choi DK, Kwon O, et al. The association between obesity and the Nocturia in the U.S. population. International Neurourology Journal. 2019;**23**(2):169-176

[90] Hagovska M, Svihra J, Bukova A, Horbacz A, Drackova D, Luptak J, et al. The relationship between overweight and overactive bladder symptoms. Obesity Facts. 2020;**13**(3):297-306

[91] Osborn DJ, Strain M, Gomelsky A, Rothschild J, Dmochowski R. Obesity and female stress urinary incontinence. Urology. 2013;**82**(4):759-763

[92] Swenson CW, Kolenic GE, Trowbridge ER, Berger MB, Lewicky-Gaupp C, Margulies RU, et al. Obesity and stress urinary incontinence in women: Compromised continence mechanism or excess

bladder pressure during cough? International Urogynecology Journal. 2017;**28**(9):1377-1385

[93] DeMarco VG, Aroor AR, Sowers JR. The pathophysiology of hypertension in patients with obesity. Nature Reviews. Endocrinology. 2014;**10**(6):364-376

[94] Kalil GZ, Haynes WG. Sympathetic nervous system in obesity-related hypertension: Mechanisms and clinical implications. Hypertension Research. 2012;**35**(1):4-16

[95] Kotsis V, Stabouli S, Papakatsika S, Rizos Z, Parati G. Mechanisms of obesity-induced hypertension. Hypertension Research. 2010;**33**(5):386-393

[96] Avelar E, Cloward TV, Walker JM, Farney RJ, Strong M, Pendleton RC, et al. Left ventricular hypertrophy in severe obesity: Interactions among blood pressure, nocturnal hypoxemia, and body mass. Hypertension. 2007;**49**(1):34-39

[97] Duflou J, Virmani R, Rabin I, Burke A, Farb A, Smialek J. Sudden death as a result of heart disease in morbid obesity. American Heart Journal. 1995;**130**(2):306-313

[98] Wolosker N, Krutman M, Kauffman P, Paula RP, Campos JR, Puech-Leao P. Effectiveness of oxybutynin for treatment of hyperhidrosis in overweight and obese patients. Revista da Associacao Medica Brasileira 1992. 2013;**59**(2):143-147

[99] Halbreich U. The etiology, biology, and evolving pathology of premenstrual syndromes. Psychoneuroendocrinology. 2003;**28**(Suppl 3):55-99

[100] McWhinney SR, Abe C, Alda M, Benedetti F, Boen E, Del Mar BC, et al. Association between body mass index and subcortical brain volumes in bipolar disorders-ENIGMA study in 2735 individuals. Molecular Psychiatry. 2021;**26**(11):6806-6819

[101] Dockray S, Susman EJ, Dorn LD. Depression, cortisol reactivity, and obesity in childhood and adolescence. The Journal of Adolescent Health. 2009;**45**(4):344-350

[102] Bianchi VE. Weight loss is a critical factor to reduce inflammation. Clinical Nutrition ESPEN. 2018;**28**:21-35

[103] Bosch-Sierra N, Grau-Del Valle C, Hermenejildo J, Hermo-Argibay A, Salazar JD, Garrido M, et al. The impact of weight loss on inflammation, oxidative stress, and mitochondrial function in subjects with obesity. Antioxidants (Basel). 2024;**13**(7):870

[104] Clamp LD, Hume DJ, Lambert EV, Kroff J. Enhanced insulin sensitivity in successful, long-term weight loss maintainers compared with matched controls with no weight loss history. Nutrition & Diabetes. 2017;**7**(6):e282

[105] Haase CL, Lopes S, Olsen AH, Satylganova A, Schnecke V, McEwan P. Weight loss and risk reduction of obesity-related outcomes in 0.5 million people: Evidence from a UK primary care database. International Journal of Obesity. 2021;**45**(6):1249-1258

[106] Ryan DH, Yockey SR. Weight loss and improvement in comorbidity: Differences at 5%, 10%, 15%, and over. Current Obesity Reports. 2017;**6**(2):187-194

[107] Magkos F, Fraterrigo G, Yoshino J, Luecking C, Kirbach K, Kelly SC, et al. Effects of moderate and subsequent progressive weight loss on metabolic function and adipose tissue biology in humans with obesity. Cell Metabolism. 2016;**23**(4):591-601

Chapter 2

Obesity in Children and Adolescents and its Impact on Mental Health

Geetanjali Sethy, Punyatoya Samal and Mamata Panda

Abstract

Obesity is a multifaceted condition that not only affects physical well-being but also has considerable psychological repercussions. Significant weight gain can result in various mental health challenges, with issues like low self-esteem and body image concerns being prevalent, alongside depression and anxiety. The stigma and discrimination encountered by individuals with obesity may exacerbate these psychological difficulties. Additionally, obesity is linked to several physical health complications, including heart disease and diabetes. It is vital to acknowledge the psychological ramifications of obesity to create effective treatment approaches that encompass both the physical and mental facets of this issue. Prompt intervention and prevention are imperative for mitigating these mental health challenges in children and adolescents with obesity. Between 1990 and 2022, the percentage of children and adolescents aged 5–19 with obesity rose fourfold from 2–8% worldwide. During the same period, the obesity rate among adults aged 18 and older more than doubled from 7–16%. This chapter examines recent statistics and articulates a problem statement concerning these two related disorders among children and adolescents.

Keywords: obesity, depression, anxiety, yoga and behavior modification, food habit

1. Introduction

The prevalence of overweight and obesity among adolescents is a significant global health concern, with alarming statistics indicating a rising trend. Worldwide, the proportion of overweight or obesity in the age group 5–19 years rose fivefold from 1975 through 2016. About 38 million children under five are overweight or obese. Projections suggest that nearly a third of the global population could be affected by 2030 [1]. The prevalence of overweight and abdominal obesity among children and adolescents globally is 21–24%. Suicide is the fourth & third leading cause of death in adolescents boys & girls respectively of age 15–19 years (**Figure 1**). Specific ethnic groups show higher rates, with obesity increasing across all pediatric ages and racial/ethnic groups, particularly in the developed countries. There is a need for effective prevention and management strategies. This condition affects physical health and has

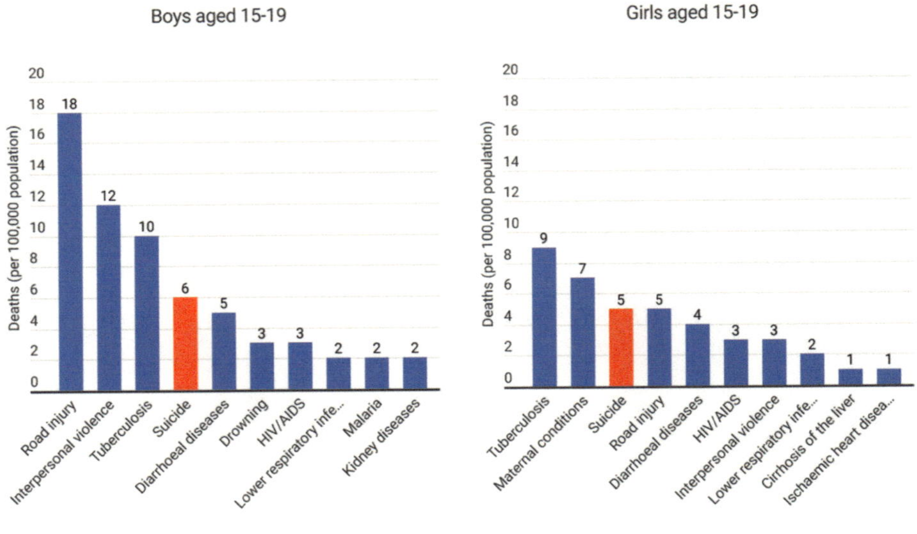

Figure 1.
Top 10 causes of death for adolescent boys and girls aged 15–19. Source: Ref. [2].

profound implications for mental and social well-being. This necessitates multifaceted approach to address its complex causes and consequences. Approximately 20.7% of children and 22.2% of adolescents are classified as obese [3]. Obesity is linked to serious health issues, including type 2 diabetes, hypertension, and psychological disorders such as depression. The relationship between obesity and mental health in children and adolescents is complex and multifaceted, with significant implications for both physical and psychological well-being [4]. Research indicates a high prevalence of depressive symptoms among youth with obesity, suggesting a strong

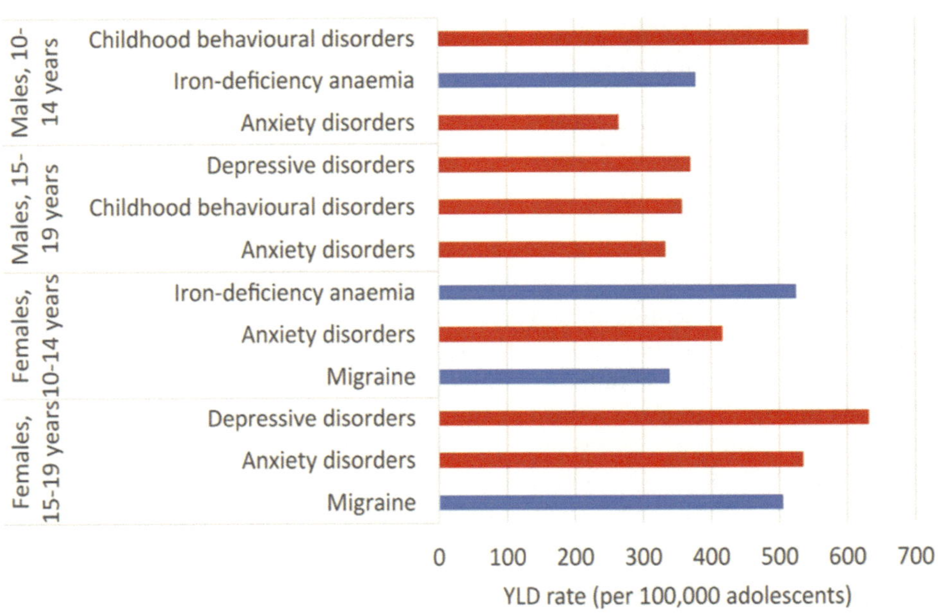

Figure 2.
Years of life lost due to diasability. Source: Ref. [5].

comorbidity between obesity and mental health issues [3]. According to Lancet the mental health issues like depression , anxiety & childhood behavioural c health problems associated with years of life lost due to disability in males and females of age 15–19 years (**Figure 2**). This interplay is influenced by various factors, including social, environmental, and genetic components. A study found that 52% of girls and 27% of boys with obesity exhibited depressive symptoms. Obesity is linked to low self-esteem and negative body image, which can exacerbate mental health issues [6]. Persistent obesity from ages 7 to 17 correlates with worsening internalizing and externalizing symptoms [7]. Conversely, reversing obesity by age 17 does not appear to negatively impact mental health, indicating potential for recovery.

2. Global statistics

The global prevalence of overweight and obesity among children and adolescents has increased significantly. In developed countries, obesity rates among adolescents are particularly high, with estimates of 21–24% prevalence.

2.1 Country-specific data

Recent studies indicate that the overall prevalence of obesity in this demographic is approximately 8.5%, with rates ranging from 0.4% in Vanuatu to 28.4% in Puerto Rico. This variation is influenced by factors such as economic status, urbanization, and lifestyle changes. In India, the prevalence of overweight among adolescents is reported at 4.8%, with urban areas showing higher rates. In another study from India, the prevalence of overweight and obesity among adolescents was found to be 7 and 5.4%, respectively [8].

In Nepal, a study found a prevalence of 6.38% among adolescents, linked to lifestyle factors such as physical inactivity and high-calorie diets [9]. High-income countries generally report higher obesity rates, correlating with higher Human Development Index scores [10]. Indonesia reports obesity rates of 10% for children aged 5 to 17 years [11]. Conversely, while the focus is often on high-income countries, low- and middle-income nations are experiencing rising obesity rates due to urbanization and dietary shifts, highlighting the need for targeted interventions globally.

The relationship between obesity and mental health issues in children and adolescents varies significantly across different countries, as evidenced by recent studies. In the UK, obesity trajectories from ages 7 to 17 are linked to worsening mental health, particularly internalizing symptoms, while obesity reversal does not negatively impact mental health outcomes [12]. In Mexico, a systematic review indicates that children who are overweight or obese are more likely to experience depression, especially among females, although the link to anxiety remains unclear. United Kingdom reports that obesity persistence correlates with increased internalizing symptoms at age 17. Reversal of obesity does not lead to negative mental health outcomes. Similarly studies from Korea reveal perceived weight status significantly affecting mental health, with misperceptions leading to increased depressive symptoms and stress [13].

Multinational analysis shows obesity is linked to higher rates of anxiety and depression, with adolescents experiencing pain more frequently [14].

Conversely, while obesity is often associated with mental health issues, some studies suggest that the impact of perceived weight status may be more significant than actual weight, indicating a complex interplay between self-image and mental health outcomes.

Despite these concerning trends, some argue that the focus on obesity may overshadow other pressing health issues, such as undernutrition and mental health challenges, which also require urgent attention in adolescent populations.

3. Why adolescents are so vulnerable?

3.1 Normal psychosocial development of adolescents

According to WHO, mental health is defined as a state of well-being in which every individual recognizes their own potential, can manage the normal stresses of life, works productively and efficiently, and is able to contribute to their community. Adolescence is a time marked by significant changes in physical, sexual, and brain development. During this stage, individuals face both opportunities and vulnerabilities that can influence their psychosocial growth. There is an interplay between biological and environmental factors. While biological changes may heighten certain behavioral tendencies, actual behavior is ultimately shaped by the social context.

3.2 Key domains of psychosocial development

1. Emotional development: Children learn to recognize and manage their emotions, which is foundational for healthy relationships and self-regulation [15].

2. Social development: Interaction with peers and family fosters social skills, including cooperation, empathy, and conflict resolution

3. Cognitive development: Cognitive skills evolve, enabling children to think critically and solve problems, which is essential for adapting to various life situations.

3.3 Other influences on development

- Environmental factors: The child's upbringing, cultural context, and peer relationships play a significant role in shaping psychosocial skills.

3.4 Physiology of brain development

There is a window of opportunity between childhood and adolescent brain development. Childhood brain development is characterized by fastest development of neural connexions, which is influenced by all modifiable factors such as nutrition, stimulation, and protection. However, adolescent brain development is characterized by neural plasticity, which means the brain recognizes and adjusts its neural connexions in response to environmental stimuli. Hence, adolescent brain development is influenced by some modifiable as well as no modifiable factors such as experience, environment, and genetics.

3.5 Adolescent brain: A second window of opportunity!

As we know first 2–3 years of life is known as the first window of opportunity (1000 days of life) (**Figure 3**). Much has been studied now and everyone is aware of

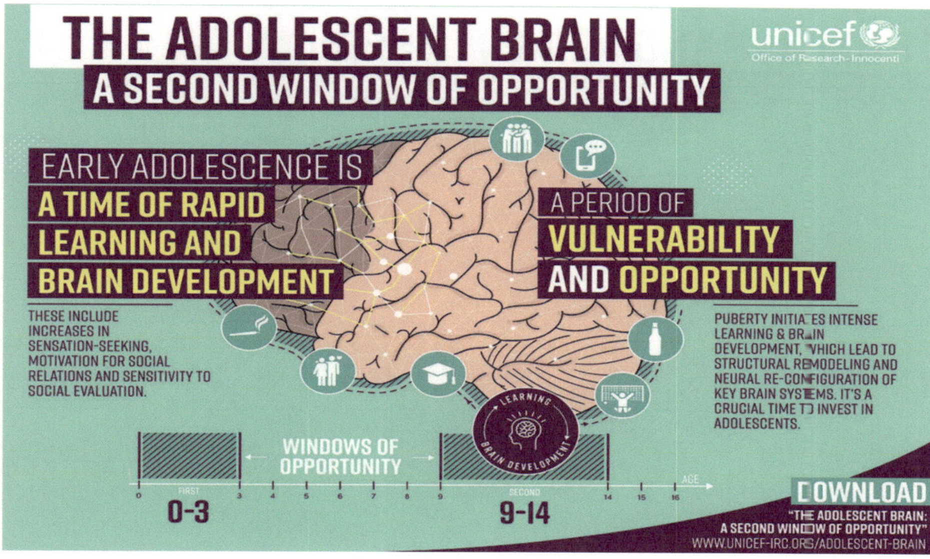

Figure 3.
Second window of opportunity: The adolescent brain. Source: https://www.unicef-irc.org/adolescent-brain.

this phase of life. But not many are aware of the second window of opportunity which is the adolescent period, the age of 9–14 years. It is crucial to support the adolescent brain to foster positive cycles and prevent negative ones, which can hinder brain development. **Figure 4** depicts some of the important positive & negative spirals of adolescent brain development. Early adolescence is a time of rapid learning and brain development. This includes sensation seeking, motivation for social relations, and sensitivity to social evaluation.

Puberty triggers significant learning and development in the brain. Structural changes and neural reorganization occur during this stage. Adolescent brain development involves both positive and negative cycles. It is crucial to support the adolescent brain to foster positive cycles and prevent negative ones, which can hinder brain development. Brain maturation begins with growth in childhood and transitions into a pruning phase during adolescence, continuing through young adulthood.

These are the brain areas involved in psychosocial development.

1. Pre-frontal cortex—reasoning and learning

2. Visual cortex/amygdala—basic memory

3. Hippocampus—emotional regulation

4. White matter connectivity—emotion and social processing

Adolescents undergo significant psychosocial development characterized by the establishment of identity, autonomy, and social relationships. This period is marked by rapid changes influenced by biological, psychological, and social factors that are crucial for understanding their behavior and interactions. The following sections outline key aspects of normal psychosocial development in adolescents.

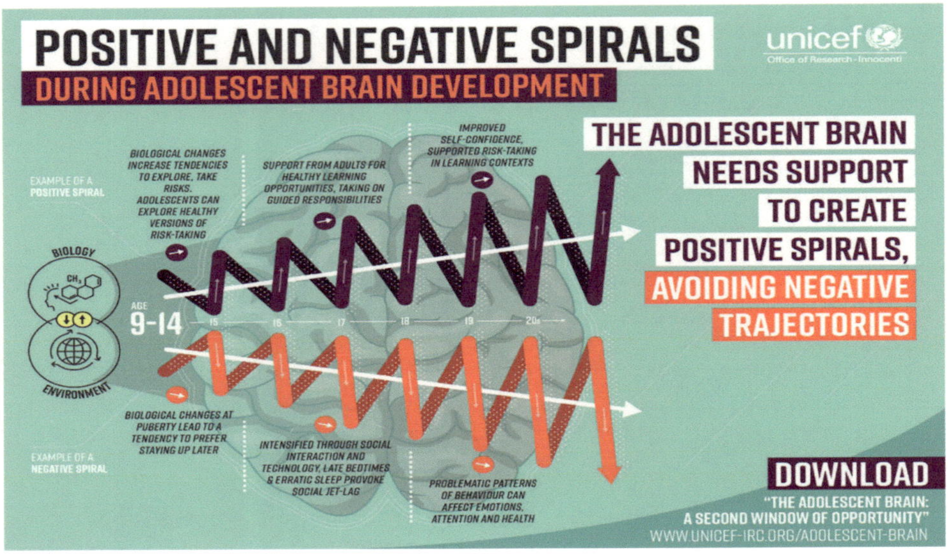

Figure 4.
Spirals affecting adolescent brain development. Source: https://www.unicef-irc.org/adolescent-brain.

3.6 Identity formation

Adolescents strive to establish a personal identity, often exploring different roles and beliefs. This process is influenced by peer interactions and parental guidance, shaping their self-concept and social identity.

3.7 Autonomy and independence

A critical developmental task is achieving autonomy from parents, which involves making independent decisions and taking responsibility for actions. This quest for independence can lead to risk-taking behaviors, as adolescents test boundaries and seek new experiences.

3.8 Social relationships

Peer relationships become increasingly important, providing emotional support and a sense of belonging [16]. Romantic relationships also emerge, contributing to emotional development and social skills.

While the majority of adolescents navigate these developmental tasks successfully, some may experience deviations due to environmental factors, such as low parental monitoring or high-risk peer influences, which can lead to psychosocial challenges such as anxiety or substance abuse [17].

Understanding these dynamics is essential for supporting healthy adolescent development.

3.9 Socioeconomic and environmental influences

Factors such as food deserts and parental influence play critical roles in the bidirectional relationship between obesity and mental health. Community-level interventions are essential for addressing these intertwined issues.

4. Relationship between obesity and mental health

While the evidence strongly supports the link between obesity and mental health challenges, it is also important to consider that not all children with obesity experience mental health issues, indicating variability in individual resilience and environmental support.

Obesity significantly impacts mental health, contributing to various psychological disorders and diminished well-being. Research indicates that higher adiposity is causally linked to increased odds of depression and lower well-being scores, with a one standard deviation increase in BMI correlating with a 50% higher likelihood of current depression [18]. Additionally, obesity is associated with chronic mental disorders, with individuals having a BMI ≥ 30 showing a 2.32 times higher probability of such conditions.The psychosocial effects, including weight stigma and discrimination, further exacerbate mental health issues, leading to increased psychological distress [19].

Key associations

1. Depression and well-being: Higher BMI correlates with increased depression and decreased well-being [18, 20].

2. Chronic mental disorders: Obesity significantly raises the risk of chronic mental health issues

3. Psychosocial factors: Weight stigma contributes to negative self-perception and mental health decline [19].

4. Socioeconomic and environmental factors: Factors such as food deserts and parental influence significantly affect both obesity and mental health outcomes [21, 22]. Community-level interventions are essential for addressing these intertwined issues.

5. Association with depression: A study found that 52% of girls and 27% of boys with obesity exhibited depressive symptoms, highlighting a strong comorbidity between obesity and mental health issues. The persistence of obesity from childhood into adolescence correlates with worsening internalizing symptoms, such as anxiety and depression, by age 17 years.

Body image and self-esteem: Children with obesity report significantly higher odds of negative body image and lower self-esteem compared to their peer. The stigma associated with obesity can lead to social isolation and further exacerbate mental health issues, creating a vicious cycle.

4.1 Bidirectional relationship

4.1.1 Chicken or egg?

Conversely, poor mental health can also lead to obesity, as individuals may engage in unhealthy behaviors such as smoking, which can exacerbate weight gain This bidirectional relationship highlights the complexity of obesity and mental health interactions. While the evidence strongly supports the link between obesity and mental health challenges, it is also important to consider that not all children with obesity experience mental health issues, suggesting a need for tailored interventions that address individual circumstances. The relationship between obesity and mental health is bidirectional; mental health issues can contribute to unhealthy eating habits, while obesity can lead to psychological distress.

Conversely, some studies suggest that interventions targeting obesity can improve mental health outcomes, indicating that addressing physical health may also alleviate psychological burdens. This highlights the importance of integrated treatment approaches for obesity and mental health in children and adolescents.

https://github.com/citation-style-language/styles/blob/master/vancouver-brackets.csl

Obesity in children and adolescents has emerged as a critical global health issue, with prevalence rates rising dramatically over the past few decades. The World Health Organization reported an increase from 4% in 1975 to over 18% in 2016, highlighting the urgent need for effective prevention and management strategies. This condition not only affects physical health but also has profound implications for mental and social well-being, necessitating a multifaceted approach to address its complex causes and consequences.

4.1.2 Prevalence and health implications

- Approximately 20.7% of children and 22.2% of adolescents are classified having obesity. Obesity is linked to serious health issues, including type 2 diabetes, hypertension, and psychological disorders such as depression.

4.1.3 Causes of obesity

- Contributing factors include genetic predisposition, dietary habits, physical inactivity, and socioeconomic influences.

- A significant portion of children engage in sedentary behaviors, with many not participating in regular physical activity.

5. Mental health and obesity: Cause, effect, and associations

It has been proven in research that obesity is related to mental health issues in both adults and children. The incidence of mental health issues, both diagnosed conditions and psychosocial issues, is greater in obese individuals. The temporal relationship between two remains yet to be established yet we have some evidence in support of the relationship,

5.1 Does obesity breed mental health issues: What we know so far?

5.1.1 Sociobehavioral

Obesity in childhood and adolescence has widespread effect on psychosocial development of the individual. With myriads of changes happening in physical, mental, emotional, and social aspects of life during adolescence, the individual is highly susceptible toward developing mental health issues. The children with obesity are subjected to constant picking, teasing, derogatory comments, and bullying. Both obesity and psychiatric illness are independently associated with stigma, teasing, and bullying [23, 24]. This in turn produces a negative self-image, which later may manifest clinically diagnosed depressive symptoms. Compared to their peers, adolescents with obesity report more internalized weight stigma, body dissatisfaction, and lower self-esteem, which further affect their mental health [23, 25]. Negative self-body image, bullying, and weight-biased peer interactions, with negative school experiences, disrupt the psychosocial development of a child. Obesity in preadolescent youth has been found to be predictive of bullying or weight-based victimization. Childhood and adolescent obesity has been also linked with comorbidities such as metabolic syndrome, type 2 diabetes, hypertension, dyslipidemia, disordered sleep, and orthopedic problems in adult life with quiet early onset [26–28]. Such chronic health conditions lead to repeated hospital visits, and doctor appointments grossly affect health-adjusted quality of life (QALY) leading to missed schools, inadequate playtime, and social interaction, which add to an already psychosocially disturbed child [29, 30]. Adolescents with obesity have shown to have poor suboptimal healthcare and less engagement with health behaviors [31, 32]. Healthcare personnel find it difficult to engage with such patients and there is poor adherence to treatment and follow-up. Adolescents with obesity tend to have more of both internalizing (depression, anxiety) and externalizing (hyperactivity, aggression) behaviors [28].

5.1.2 Pathophysiological

Obesity's pathophysiology involves genetics, epigenetics, environmental factors, social influences, and lifestyle choices. The rising incidence of obesity among younger populations in the recent decades has been linked to the consumption of high-fat, palatable foods, and a sedentary lifestyle. Research indicates that high-fat diets trigger the release of proinflammatory cytokines, such as TNF-α and interleukin (IL-1β), in the hypothalamus. This hypothalamic inflammation disrupts central energy regulation, as well as insulin secretion and sensitivity. This localized inflammatory response, known as "neuroinflammation," creates an imbalance between microglial cells and astrocytes, impacting neurotransmitter metabolism and the production of growth factors. Consequently, plasticity processes, including synaptic production, remodeling, and neurogenesis, are hindered, particularly in crucial areas such as the hypothalamus, hippocampus, and prefrontal cortex, termed as "neuroprogression." Ultimately, neurodegenerative processes may develop, leading to irreversible lesions (like gliotic scars) and, crucially, the loss of neural cells in the brain. These structural changes help explain why obesity increases the risk of psychiatric disorders, including mood disorders, and establish a theoretical framework for understanding the connection between weight status and neuropsychological functions, such as cognitive/executive abilities and emotion regulation [33, 34]. The hippocampus plays a vital role in cognition, memory (both long and short term), and learning. Conditions associated with obesity, such as diabetes, hypertension, obstructive sleep apnea (OSA), and cardiovascular diseases, negatively impact brain volume, particularly in the hippocampus [35]. Excessive nutrition during early life has been shown to lead to brain insulin resistance and subsequent hippocampal atrophy, resulting in functional loss that contributes to cognitive decline and abnormal eating habits later in life, perpetuating a cycle of overeating, obesity, and adverse mental health effects [36].

5.1.3 Genetics

Genetics have been attributed to childhood and adolescent obesity especially having severe obesity (BMI ≥120% of 95th centile for age and sex), eary-onset obesity (before age of 5 years), hyperphagia, and family history of consanguinity with developmental and physical abnormalities of genetic syndromes [37]. Syndromic forms of obesity include Prader-Willi syndrome, Alström syndrome, Brdet-Biedel syndrome, Smith-Maegins syndrome, Cohen syndrome, Beckwith-Weidman syndrome, and many more. Monogenetic forms include mostly various forms of leptin pathway deficiency, MC4R deficiency, proprotein subtilisin or kexin type 1 deficiency, SRC1 deficiency, brain-derived neurotrophic factor (BDNF) deficiency, etc. [37]. Mediators of leptin pathway are part of other signaling pathways involved in neurological development and neurological abnormalities, and defects in the Leptin pathway, such as executive function impairments and developmental delays, are notable. The melanocortin-4 receptor (MC4R) defect correlates with a high incidence of attention-deficit/hyperactivity disorder (ADHD) [38, 39]. Variants of the BDNF gene are linked to hyperphagia and severe early-onset obesity, as well as cognitive impairments and altered pain perception [40–42]. Prader-Willi syndrome features include intellectual disability, pain insensitivity, aggressive behavior, and temper tantrums. Bardet-Biedl syndrome is associated with obsessive-compulsive disorder and emotional outbursts. Patients with Smith-Magenis syndrome exhibit self-injurious behavior, intellectual disabilities, and stereotyped behaviors, particularly spasmodic upper-body self-hugging [43]. As the various studies show, genetics involved in early onset obesity are involved in neurodevelopmental pathways indicating correlation between obesity and evolution of mental health conditions.

5.2 Can mental health conditions propagate obesity: Assumptions and facts

The prevalence of adolescent mental health conditions have increased many fold over last few years [44]. It is because of changing socioeconomic and environmental standards and also has better accessibility to health care facilities. As discussed above, mental health issues and obesity have a bidirectional relationship [45]. Studies have identified internalizing (i.e., depression) and externalizing (i.e., hyperactivity, aggression) behaviors during middle childhood, respectively, as predictors of obesity in late adolescence and young adulthood [46, 47]. Other studies have suggested that childhood hyperactivity and inattention place a person at increased risk for obesity later in life [48]. Many study findings support the hypothesis that depression is an independent predictor of obesity [49, 50]. Adolescents with psychiatric disorders tend to report unhealthier dietary and physical activity behaviors such as higher total energy intake and higher intake of energy-dense and processed foods [51]. Adolescent females with high depressive symptoms are two times more likely to develop overeating and binge eating as compared to their normal counterparts [52]. Adolescents with bipolar disorder report worse nutrition and eating habits in comparison with their healthy counterparts [53]. Studies also reveal association between depression and lower levels of physical activity [54] and higher sedentary behaviors [55]. Lack of motivation, internalized behavioral patterns, and perceived body image issues all lead to a vicious cycle while a teen does not want engage in healthy lifestyles such as exercise and dietary controls but rather tend to overeat. The term "emotional eating" which refers to binge-eating episodes with changes in emotional status as described in eating disorders is a major contributing factor to adolescent obesity [56]. Total screen time is related to higher depressive symptoms in adolescents with overweight and obesity [57]. The rampant use of electronic device in present time has been identified as a contributing factor for the development of psychiatric disorders [58]. Children glued to their phone screens not only impact their mental health, but promote sedentary lifestyle, which in turn causes excessive weight gain.

Adolescents having psychiatric disorders are treated with psychiatric medications, which have weight gain as a major side effect [59]. Antipsychotics that are used to treat bipolar and schizophrenia-spectrum disorders have been associated with greater weight gain relative to placebo or to not taking antipsychotics in young patients [60]. In particular, second-generation antipsychotics can cause significant and rapid weight gain compared to first-generation antipsychotics [60]. Earlier use of antipsychotics during childhood and adolescence results in a longer lifetime exposure to their adverse effects leading to cumulative effect. Adolescents appear be at higher risk for antipsychotic-induced weight gain in comparison with adults [61]. Rate of weight is maximum in the beginning of starting an antipsychotic, usually first 3 to 6 months, and then continues at a constant rate throughout [62]. Antipsychotic drugs have different weight gain propensities. Drugs such as olanzepine and clozapine have adverse weight gain potential [63, 64]. Evidence suggests a correlation between antipsychotic-induced weight gain and therapeutic benefit for psychiatric illness. Some studies suggest that weight gain was associated with greater reductions in symptoms in psychiatric illness on use of the antipsychotics [59, 65]. This is an interesting aspect that needs further research and evidence. It is seen that the neurotransmitters such as histamine H1 (H1), serotonin 2A/2C (5-HT2A/C), and dopamine D1/D2/D3 receptors, which are implicated in the therapeutic actions of antipsychotics, are involved in weight regulation mechanisms [66]. However, drugs such as lithium, carbamazepine, or valproic acid derivatives are used as mood stabilizers and serotonin reuptake inhibitors (SSRIs) used in depression evidence is more inconsistent among adolescents regarding weight gain tendencies.

We have previously discussed how genetics and biologic pathways involved in obesity can cause mental health issues. The same holds good for other way around too. A study suggests about 12% of the genetic component implicated in depression is the same as that of obesity [67]. Genes such as FTO, POMC, ITIH4, TLR4, BDNF, and CREB1 show association with both obesity and various psychiatric disorders [68]. Another study demonstrated that participants with major depressive disorder who reported increased appetite/weight during a depressive episode carried higher genetic risk for elevated BMI and inflammatory markers [69]. Various biological mechanisms proposed for correlating mental disorders and obesity include altered circadian rhythms [70], dysregulated hypothalamic-pituitary-adrenocortical axis leading to inflammation, imbalanced hormones, and neurotransmitters [71, 72].

6. Obesity-associated major psychiatric comorbidities

6.1 Depression

Depression is classified as a mood disorder. Mood disorder consists of psychiatric symptoms characterized by deficit in emotional self-regulation. Depressive symptoms consist of disturbance of sleep, appetite and activity, thoughts of worthlessness or guilt, impaired concentration, low productivity and energy, and suicidal thoughts or actions. Such adolescents show sudden withdrawal from social activity and tend to cope up in their personal space isolating from outside world. Overeating may be seen with minimal physical activity level. They tend to either sleep a lot or find it difficult to sleep. Studies have shown that relationships between obesity and depression may be bidirectional. Youths having obesity tend to have higher occurrence of obesity as compared to normal weight peers [73]. It has been seen that obesity increases severity of depressive symptoms among youngsters [73]. The association between depression causing obesity appears to be stronger than obesity causing depression as per studies [74]. The relationship between depression and obesity is stronger among females than males [75]. Individuals with obesity have higher chance of having suicidal thoughts and a greater risk of premature death by suicide thoughts too [76, 77]. Obesity as a contributor of depression is multidimensional. The social and emotional implications of obesity over an adolescent mental health are variable but long-lasting. Adolescents having obesity must be screened for obesity even in the absence of clinical symptoms and appropriate intervention must be started as early as possible.

6.2 Bipolar disorder

Bipolar disorder is classified under mood disorders. Bipolar disorder comprises of episodes of mania alternating with depressive moods. Manic episode refers to period of abnormally and persistently elevated expansive or irritable mood with increased goal-directed activities with associated elevated self-esteem, decreased need for sleep, flight of ideas, distractibility, more goal-directed activities or purposeless non-goal-directed activities, or involvement in high potential risky activities, which may cause painful experiences (DSM-5). The manic episodes alter with depression symptoms for various periods of time. There are various groups of bipolar disorders based on duration and type of manic and depressive episodes. Patients with bipolar disorder have increased risk of overweight, obesity, and pathologic eating, in both adults and adolescents [78–80]. Bipolar disorder especially type II presents with atypical depressive symptoms types such as hyperphagia and hypersomnia may cause excessive weight gain [81, 82]. Obesity is correlated with the increased bipolar disorder severity [83, 84] including suicidal behavior self-injury [85]. As discussed previously, some drugs like atypical antipsychotics such as olanzapine and clozapine used to treat bipolar disorder have weight gain potential. Patients with bipolar disorder and obesity are difficult to treat as psychotropic drugs used in its management can induce further weight gain, seen particularly in case of atypical antipsychotics, and their combination with mood stabilizers provides a challenging scenario [79]. Association of bipolar disorder with eating disorder, in particular binge eating disorder, leads to a more severe form of obesity, making treatment difficult for both patient and physician [86–88].

6.3 Eating disorders

Eating disorders are the disorders associated with dysfuctional eating patterns associated with cognitive and emotional dysregulation. Eating disorders most commonly associated with obesity is binge eating disorder (BED). BED refers to recurrent episodes of episodes of excessive and uncontrolled eating to the point of uncontrollable and painful fullness. It is different from another common eating disorder Bulimia nervosa (BN), which is characterized by brief periods of excessive eating followed by compensatory behaviors such as self-induced purging, laxative ad diuretic use, exercising. BED is highly associated with obesity associated with BN is to a lesser extent owing to the weight-reducing activities associated with AN [89]. As discussed previously, obesity is linked with dysregulation in the leptin pathway, which affects the hypothalamic mechanisms of energy homeostasis. Additionally, it disrupts the reward and emotional circuits in the amygdala, leading to disordered eating behaviors [90, 91]. The terms "food addiction" can be associated with obesity and eating disorders (EDs), which stem from varied disorganization in eating habits and deficits in the regulation of appetite, reward, and emotions localized to the dopaminergic pathways of the mesolimbic system [91–98]. The psychological basis of binge eating disorder (BED) is thought to be an acquired behavioral strategy aimed at coping with adverse situations that the individual cannot manage otherwise [99]. Emotional eating, defined as a form of dysregulated eating where individuals feel compelled to eat in reaction to stressful situations or intense negative emotions, shows a strong connection to BED [100]. Managing BED alongside comorbid obesity is particularly challenging, as patients with BED tend to exhibit a poorer metabolic profile compared to those without BED and are at a higher risk for conditions such as type 2 diabetes mellitus and fatty liver disease [101–104]. Furthermore, the combination of BED and obesity increases the likelihood of developing psychiatric comorbidities, including anxiety and mood disorders [105]. Therefore, treating eating disorders and obesity presents a significant challenge for healthcare professionals.

6.4 ADHD

Attention-deficit/hyperactivity disorder (ADHD) characterized by cardinal symptoms of inattentiveness, hyperactivity, and impulsivity is one of the most common neurobehavioral problems of growing up. It widely affects children of school-going age and carries over into adulthood. The possible connection between obesity and ADHD has been widely studied and it appears to be extensive and multi-dimensional. There is a high probability of attention-deficit/hyperactivity disorder (ADHD) in children and adolescents with high BMI [106]. Studies show a higher body mass index (BMI) increases the risk of developing ADHD [107]. The probable structural and neurobiological connection between obesity and ADHD involves dysregulation in common brain dopaminergic reward pathways, emotion regulation processes, and executive functions [108]. Inattention in children and adolescents suffering from ADHD leads to difficulty in controlling their overeating tendencies. The dysregulated dopaminergic reward system makes them prone to be addicted to fatty, calorie rich food as a means of achieving instant gratification, which is a common finding in ADHD. Emotional dysfunction may manifest as impulsive episodes of uncontrolled overeating. Similarly, dysregulated planning and organization functions observed in ADHD lead to difficulties in controlling eating behavior and inattention may cause lack of awareness of hunger and satiety, which leads to uncontrolled eating [109]. Patients with ADHD often suffer from early insomnia due to delayed release of melatonin [110], and lack of enough sleep has been described as one of underlying mechanism in the development of obesity [111]. ADHD impacts treatment of obesity as impulsivity and inattention makes it difficult for compliance for treatment. However, it has been shown that treatment of ADHD in childhood reduces risk of obesity [112]. This may be explained as reduction in cardinal symptoms of ADHD occurs, and improvement in executive functions leads to better compliance to diet and lifestyle changes [107].

7. Management strategies

7.1 Therapeutic interventions

- Group psychotherapy can enhance psychosocial development by providing a supportive environment for children to explore their feelings and social interactions [113]
- Effective management requires personalized interventions, including dietary modifications, increased physical activity, and behavioral therapy
- Pharmacological options and bariatric surgery may be considered for severe cases, particularly in adolescents

Despite the alarming rise in childhood obesity, some argue that societal changes, such as increased awareness and community-based interventions, may help reverse this trend. However, the complexity of obesity necessitates ongoing research and tailored strategies to ensure effective prevention and treatment.

Normal psychosocial development in children encompasses a range of changes that occur from infancy through adolescence, significantly influenced by their environment and relationships. This development is crucial for children to effectively interact with their surroundings and build essential life skills. Key aspects of this process include emotional, social, and cognitive growth, which are interrelated and shaped by both intrinsic factors and external influences.

While the focus is often on typical development, it is important to recognize that variations exist due to individual differences and external circumstances. Understanding these nuances can help caregivers and professionals better support children's psychosocial growth.

7.2 Prevention and management

Overweight and obesity can be prevented. Effective prevention is crucial for addressing the growing global epidemic. Initiatives must begin as early as the preconception period.

Key strategies include:

- Ensuring appropriate weight gain during pregnancy;
- Practicing exclusive breastfeeding for the first 6 months after birth and continuing breastfeeding until 24 months or longer;
- Modifying children's behaviors toward healthy eating, physical activity, sedentary habits, and sleep, irrespective of their current weight status;
- Reducing screen time;
- Limiting the intake of sugary beverages and energy-dense foods while encouraging healthy eating practices;
- Leading a healthy lifestyle (balanced diet, regular physical activity, adequate sleep, and avoiding tobacco and alcohol, as well as managing emotions);

- Minimizing energy intake from fats and sugars while increasing the consumption of fruits, vegetables, legumes, whole grains, and nuts; and
- Participating in consistent physical activity.

7.3 Role of health practitioners

- Measure children's weight and height during every visit to health facilities;
- Offer guidance on healthy diets and lifestyles;
- Upon diagnosing obesity, deliver comprehensive prevention and management services focused on healthy eating, physical activity, as well as medical and surgical options; and
- Track other non-communicable disease risk factors (blood glucose, lipids, and blood pressure) and evaluate for comorbidities and disabilities, including mental health issues.

7.4 Role of community and administration

Dietary and physical activity patterns are largely influenced by environmental and societal factors that restrict personal choices. Combating obesity is a collective societal responsibility, and successful solutions must cultivate environments and communities that normalize healthy eating and regular physical activity as accessible and affordable aspects of daily life.

To stop the rise in obesity, it is essential to adopt multisectoral strategies that encompass food production, marketing, pricing, and additional efforts focused on addressing broader health determinants such as poverty reduction and urban development.

Such policies and actions include:

- Structural, fiscal, and regulatory initiatives aimed at establishing healthy food environments that make nutritious options available, accessible, and appealing; and
- Health sector strategies are designed and equipped to identify risks, prevent, manage, and treat diseases. These actions should build on and integrate with broader efforts to tackle non-communicable diseases (NCDs) and enhance health systems through a primary health care framework.

The food industry can significantly contribute to promoting healthy diets by following:

- Reducing the fat, sugar, and salt content in processed foods.
- Ensuring consumers have access to healthy and nutritious food.
- Banning or at least restricting the promotion of foods high in salt, sugar, and fat.

- Making healthy food choices readily available in the workplace.
- Encouraging regular physical activity within the workplace.

8. Conclusions

Obesity and mental health issues are widespread and considered significant health challenges. Over the past few decades, obesity rates have increased by more than 6%, and over 12% of children and adolescents experience psychiatric disorders. Prioritizing self-care is crucial for developing resilience, which helps to ensure that our children's mental and physical health remains robust in facing challenges. Encouraging children to concentrate on their well-being is essential. Engaging them in activities that promote joy and relaxation effectively reduces the risks related to obesity and mental health disorders. The basis for preventing and managing these interrelated conditions consists of structured physical exercise, play therapy, and a nutritious diet.

Conflict of interests

The authors declare no conflict of interest.

Author details

Geetanjali Sethy[1*], Punyatoya Samal[1] and Mamata Panda[2]

1 SCB Medical College and Hospital, Cuttack, Odisha, India

2 Care Group of Hospitals, Bhubaneswar, Odisha, India

*Address all correspondence to: geetanjalisethy@gmail.com

References

[1] Mamatkhuzhaeva G, Arzikulov A. Prevention of obesity In children and adolescents and modern technologies of medical rehabilitation. International Journal of Scientific Pediatrics. 2024;**3**(6):642-647

[2] Guthold R et al. The top global causes of adolescent mortality and morbidity by age and sex. Journal of Adolescent Health. 2019;**69**(4):540

[3] Matson KL, Fenn NE 3rd. Obesity management in the pediatric patient. American Journal of Health-System Pharmacy. 17 Apr 2025;**82**(8):392-402. DOI: 10.1093/ajhp/zxae236

[4] Henriques J, Afreixo V, Unterrainer H, Senra H. Psychological mediators of the association between obesity and symptoms of depression, anxiety, and stress. Neuropsychobiology. 2025;**84**(1):26-37. DOI: 10.1159/000542767. Epub 2024 Nov 25

[5] Kyu HH et al. Global, regional, and national disability-adjusted life-years (DALYs) for 359 diseases and injuries and healthy life expectancy (HALE) for 195 countries and territories, 1990-2017: A systematic analysis for the global burden of disease study 2017. The Lancet. 2018;**392**(10159):1859-1922

[6] Iversen KD, Pedersen TP, Rasmussen M, Hansen MBL, Roikjer BH, Teilmann G. Mental health and BMI in children and adolescents during one year in obesity treatment. BMC Pediatrics. 2024;**24**:406. DOI: 10.1186/s12887-024-04835-7

[7] Putra IGNE, Daly M, Sutin A, Steptoe A, Scholes S, Robinson E. Obesity, psychological well-being related measures, and risk of seven non-communicable diseases: Evidence from longitudinal studies of UK and US older adults. International Journal of Obesity. 2024;**48**(9):1283-1291

[8] Sethi V, Bassi S, Bahl D, Kumar A, Choedon T, Bhatia N, et al. Prevalence of overweight and obesity and associated demographic and health factors in India: Findings from comprehensive National Nutrition Survey (CNNS). Pediatric Obesity. Apr 2024;**19**(4):e13092. DOI: 10.1111/ijpo.13092. Epub 2024 Feb 7

[9] Gautam N, Rahman MM, Hashmi R, Lim A, Khanam R. Socioeconomic inequalities in child and adolescent mental health in Australia: The role of parenting style and parents' relationships. Child and Adolescent Psychiatry and Mental Health. 2024;**18**(1):28. DOI: 10.1186/s13034-024-00719-x

[10] Zhang X, Liu J, Ni Y, et al. Global prevalence of overweight and obesity in children and adolescents: A systematic review and meta-analysis. JAMA Pediatrics. 2024;**178**(8):800-813. DOI: 10.1001/jamapediatrics.2024.1576

[11] Akbar Z, Naeem S, Javed S, et al. Risk factors of overweight and obesity in childhood and adolescence in Pakistan, a systematic review. Discover Public Health. 2025;**22**:75. DOI: 10.1186/s12982-025-00465-1

[12] Ngurah Edi Putra IG, Daly M, Robinson E. Childhood obesity trajectories and adolescent mental health: A UK cohort study. Pediatric Obesity. 2025;**20**(3):e13206. DOI: 10.1111/ijpo.13206

[13] Choi Y, Hong J. Association between weight status and mental

health among Korean adolescents: A Nationwide cross-sectional study. Children. 2023;**10**(4):620. DOI: 10.3390/children10040620

[14] Barnard-Kelly K, Whicher CA, Price HC, et al. Liraglutide and the management of overweight and obesity in people with severe mental illness: Qualitative sub-study. BMC Psychiatry. 2022;**22**:21. DOI: 10.1186/s12888-021-03666-5

[15] Orenstein GA, Lewis L. Erikson's Stages of Psychosocial Development. Treasure Island (FL): StatPearls Publishing; 2025. Available from: https://www.ncbi.nlm.nih.gov/books/NBK556096/

[16] Gaete J, Martinez V, Fritsch R, et al. Indicated school-based intervention to improve depressive symptoms among at risk Chilean adolescents: A randomized controlled trial. BMC Psychiatry. 2016;**16**:276. DOI: 10.1186/s12888-016-0985-4

[17] Evans M, Fisher EB. Social isolation and mental health: The role of nondirective and directive social support. Community Mental Health Journal. 2022;**58**:20-40. DOI: 10.1007/s10597-021-00787-9

[18] Casanova F, O'Loughlin J, Martin S, Beaumont RN, Wood AR, Watkins ER, et al. Higher adiposity and mental health: Causal inference using Mendelian randomization. Human Molecular Genetics. 2021;**30**(24):2371-2382. DOI: 10.1093/hmg/ddab204

[19] Melamed OC, Selby P, Taylor VH. Mental health and obesity during the COVID-19 pandemic. Current Obesity Reports. 2022;**11**:23-31. DOI: 10.1007/s13679-021-00466-6

[20] Lonergan C, Millar SR, Kabir Z. Associations between adiposity measures and depression and well-being scores: A cross-sectional analysis of middle- to older-aged adults. PLoS One. 2024;**19**(3):e0299029. DOI: 10.1371/journal.pone.0299029

[21] Kesavayuth D, Zikos V. Mental health and obesity. Applied Economic Analysis. 2024;**32**(94):41-61. DOI: 10.1108/AEA-06-2023-0212

[22] Lin M-L, Faldowski RA. The relationship of parent support and child emotional regulation to school readiness. International Journal of Environmental Research and Public Health. 2023;**20**(6):4867. DOI: 10.3390/ijerph20064867

[23] Rankin J, Matthews L, Cobley S, Han A, Sanders R, Wiltshire HD, et al. Psychological consequences of childhood obesity: Psychiatric comorbidity and prevention. Adolescent Health, Medicine and Therapeutics. 2016;7:125-146

[24] Kaushik A, Kostaki E, Kyriakopoulos M. The stigma of mental illness in children and adolescents: A systematic review. Psychiatry Research. 2016;**243**:469-494

[25] Stevens SD, Herbozo S, Morrell HE, Schaefer LM, Thompson JK. Adult and childhood weight influence body image and depression through weight stigmatization. Journal of Health Psychology. 2017;**22**(8):1084-1093

[26] Sahoo K, Sahoo B, Choudhury AK, et al. Childhood obesity: Causes and consequences. Journal of Family Medicine and Primary Care. 2015;**4**(2):187-192

[27] Pulgaron ER. Childhood obesity: A review of increased risk for physical and psychological comorbidities. Clinical Therapeutics. 2013;**35**(1):A18-A32

[28] Janicke DM, Harman JS, Kelleher KJ, et al. Psychiatric diagnosis in children and adolescents with obesity-related health conditions. Journal of Developmental and Behavioral Pediatrics. 2008;**29**(4):276-284

[29] Williams JW, Canterford L, Hesketh KD, et al. Changes in body mass index and health related quality of life from childhood to adolescence. International Journal of Pediatric Obesity. 2011;**6**(2-2):e442-e448

[30] Taylor VH, Forhan M, Vigod SN, et al. The impact of obesity on quality of life. Best Practice & Research. Clinical Endocrinology & Metabolism. 2013;**27**(2):139-146

[31] Clement S, Schauman O, Graham T, Maggioni F, Evans-Lacko S, Bezborodovs N, et al. What is the impact of mental health-related stigma on help-seeking? A systematic review of quantitative and qualitative studies. Psychological Medicine. 2015;**45**(1):11-27

[32] Puhl RM, Peterson JL, Luedicke J. Parental perceptions of weight terminology that providers use with youth. Pediatrics. 2011;**128**(4):e786-e793

[33] Weiss F, Barbuti M, Carignani G, Calderone A, Santini F, Maremmani I, et al. Psychiatric aspects of obesity: A narrative review of pathophysiology and psychopathology. Journal of Clinical Medicine. 2020;**9**(8):2344. DOI: 10.3390/jcm9082344

[34] Patist CM, Stapelberg NJC, Du Toit EF, Headrick JP. The brain-adipocyte-gut network: Linking obesity and depression subtypes. Cognitive, Affective, & Behavioral Neuroscience. 2018;**18**:1121-1144

[35] Fotuhi M, Do D, Jack C. Modifiable factors that alter the size of the hippocampus with ageing. Nature Reviews. Neurology. 2012;**8**(4):189-202

[36] Kanoski SE, Zhang Y, Zheng W, Davidson TL. The effects of a high-energy diet on hippocampal function and blood-brain barrier integrity in the rat. Journal of Alzheimer's disease: JAD. 2010;**21**(1):207-219

[37] Hampl SE, Hassink SG, Skinner AC, et al. Clinical practice guideline for the evaluation and treatment of children and adolescents with obesity. Pediatrics. 2023;**151**:e2022060640

[38] Porfirio MC, Giovinazzo S, Cortese S, et al. Role of ADHD symptoms as a contributing factor to obesity in patients with MC4R mutations. Medical Hypotheses. 2015;**84**(1):4-7

[39] Agranat-Meged A, Ghanadri Y, Eisenberg I, et al. Attention deficit hyperactivity disorder in obese melanocortin-4-receptor (MC4R) deficient subjects: A newly described expression of MC4R deficiency. American Journal of Medical Genetics. Part B, Neuropsychiatric Genetics. 2008;**147B**(8):1547-1553

[40] da Fonseca ACP, Abreu GM, Palhinha L, et al. A rare potential pathogenic variant in the BDNF gene is found in a Brazilian patient with severe childhood-onset obesity. Diabetes, Metabolic Syndrome and Obesity. 2021;**14**:11-22

[41] Sonoyama T, Stadler LKJ, Zhu M, et al. Human BDNF/TrkB variants impair hippocampal synaptogenesis and associate with neurobehavioural abnormalities. Scientific Reports. 2020;**10**(1):9028

[42] Gray J, Yeo GS, Cox JJ, et al. Hyperphagia, severe obesity, impaired cognitive function, and hyperactivity

associated with functional loss of one copy of the brain-derived neurotrophic factor (BDNF) gene. Diabetes. 2006;**55**(12):3366-3371

[43] Smith ACM, Boyd KE, Brennan C, et al. Smith-Magenis syndrome. In: Adam MP, Feldman J, Mirzaa GM, et al., editors. Gene Reviews [Internet]. Seattle; Seattle (WA): University of Washington; 2001, 1993-2024

[44] Bor W, Dean AJ, Najman J, Hayatbakhsh R. Are child and adolescent mental health problems increasing in the 21st century? A systematic review. The Australian and New Zealand Journal of Psychiatry. Jul 2014;**48**(7):606-616. DOI: 10.1177/0004867414533834. Epub 2014 May 14

[45] Rajan TM, Menon V. Psychiatric disorders and obesity: A review of association studies. Journal of Postgraduate Medicine. 2017;**63**(3):182-190. DOI: 10.4103/jpgm.JPGM_712_16

[46] Epstein LH, Paluch RA, Gordy CC, et al. Decreasing sedentary behaviors in treating pediatric obesity. Archives of Pediatrics & Adolescent Medicine. 2000;**154**(3):220-226

[47] Barlow SE, Trowbridge FL, Klish WJ, et al. Treatment of child and adolescent obesity: Reports from pediatricians, pediatric nurse practitioners, and registered dieticians. Pediatrics. 2002;**110**(1):229-235

[48] White B, Nicholls D, Christie D, et al. Childhood psychological function and obesity risk across the lifecourse: Findings from the 1970 British cohort study. International Journal of Obesity. 2012;**36**(4):511-516

[49] Chang Y, Gable S. Predicting weight status stability and change from fifth grade to eighth grade: The significant role of adolescents' social-emotional well-being. The Journal of Adolescent Health. 2013;**52**(4):448-455

[50] Roberts RE, Duong HT. Obese youths are not more likely to become depressed, but depressed youths are more likely to become obese. Psychological Medicine. 2013;**43**:2143-2151. DOI: 10.1017/S0033291712002991

[51] Goodwin RD, Sourander A, Duarte CS, et al. Do mental health problems in childhood predict chronic physical conditions among males in early adulthood? Evidence from a community-based prospective study. Psychological Medicine. 2009;**39**(2):301-311

[52] O'Neil A, Quirk SE, Housden S, Brennan SL, Williams LJ, Pasco JA, et al. Relationship between diet and mental health in children and adolescents: A systematic review. American Journal of Public Health. 2014;**104**(10):e31-e42

[53] Skinner HH, Haines J, Austin SB, Field AE. A prospective study of overeating, binge eating, and depressive symptoms among adolescent and young adult women. The Journal of Adolescent Health. 2012;**50**(5):478-483

[54] Martin K, Woo J, Timmins V, Collins J, Islam A, Newton D, et al. Binge eating and emotional eating behaviors among adolescents and young adults with bipolar disorder. Journal of Affective Disorders. 2016;**195**:88-95

[55] Hoare E, Millar L, Fuller-Tyszkiewicz M, Skouteris H, Nichols M, Malakellis M, et al. Depressive symptomatology, weight status and obesogenic risk among Australian adolescents: A prospective cohort study. BMJ Open. 2016;**6**(3):e010072

[56] Castillo F, Francis L, Wylie-Rosett J, Isasi CR. Depressive symptoms are

associated with excess weight and unhealthier lifestyle behaviors in urban adolescents. Childhood Obesity. 2014;**10**(5):400-407

[57] Gianini LM, White MA, Masheb RM. Eating pathology, emotion regulation, and emotional overeating in obese adults with binge eating disorder. Eating Behaviors. 2013;**14**:309-313

[58] Goldfield GS, Murray M, Maras D, Wilson AL, Phillips P, Kenny GP, et al. Screen time is associated with depressive symptomatology among obese adolescents: A HEARTY study. European Journal of Pediatrics. 2016;**175**(7):909-919

[59] Robinson TN, Banda JA, Hale L, Lu AS, Fleming-Milici F, Calvert SL, et al. Screen media exposure and obesity in children and adolescents. Pediatrics. 2017 Nov;**140**(Suppl 2):S97-S101. DOI: 10.1542/peds.2016-1758K

[60] Raben AT, Marshe VS, Chintoh A, Gorbovskaya I, Müller DJ, Hahn M. The complex relationship between antipsychotic-induced weight gain and therapeutic benefits: A systematic review and implications for treatment. Frontiers in Neuroscience. 2017;**11**:741

[61] Pillay J, Boylan K, Carrey N, Newton A, Vandermeer B, Nuspl M, et al. First-and Second-Generation Antipsychotics in Children and Young Adults: Systematic Review Update. Rockville (MD): Agency for Healthcare Research and Quality; 2017. Contract No.: 17-EHC001-EF

[62] Ho J, Panagiotopoulos C, McCrindle B, Grisaru S, Pringsheim T, Canadian Alliance for Monitoring Effectiveness, et al. Management recommendations for metabolic complications associated with second-generation antipsychotic use in children and youth. Paediatrics & Child Health. 2011;**16**(9):575-580

[63] Bushe CJ, Slooff CJ, Haddad PM, Karagianis JL. Weight change from 3-year observational data: Findings from the worldwide schizophrenia outpatient health outcomes database. The Journal of Clinical Psychiatry. 2012;**73**(6):e749-e755

[64] Kumra S, Kranzler H, Gerbino-Rosen G, Kester HM, DeThomas C, Kafantaris V, et al. Clozapine and "high-dose" olanzapine in refractory early-onset schizophrenia: A 12-week randomized and double-blind comparison. Biological Psychiatry. 2008;**63**(5):524-529

[65] Correll CU, Manu P, Olshanskiy V, Napolitano B, Kane JM, Malhotra AK. Cardiometabolic risk of second-generation antipsychotic medications during first-time use in children and adolescents. Journal of the American Medical Association. 2009;**302**(16):1765-1773

[66] Bai YM, Lin C-C, Chen J-Y, Lin C-Y, Su T-P, Chou P. Association of initial antipsychotic response to clozapine and long-term weight gain. The American Journal of Psychiatry. 2006;**163**(7):1276-1279

[67] Afari N, Noonan C, Goldberg J, Roy-Byrne P, Schur E, Golnari G, et al. Depression and obesity: Do shared genes explain the relationship? Depression and Anxiety. 2010;**27**(9):799-806

[68] Amare AT, Schubert KO, Klingler-Hoffmann M, Cohen-Woods S, Baune BT. The genetic overlap between mood disorders and cardiometabolic diseases: A systematic review of genome wide and candidate gene studies. Translational Psychiatry. 2017;**7**(1):e1007

[69] Milaneschi Y, Lamers F, Peyrot WJ, Baune BT, Breen G, Dehghan A, et al.

Genetic association of major depression with atypical features and obesity-related immunometabolic dysregulations. JAMA Psychiatry. 2017;**74**(12):1214-1225

[70] Zelinski EL, Deibel SH, McDonald RJ. The trouble with circadian clock dysfunction: Multiple deleterious effects on the brain and body. Neuroscience and Biobehavioral Reviews. 2014;**40**:80-101

[71] Lu X-Y. The leptin hypothesis of depression: A potential link between mood disorders and obesity? Current Opinion in Pharmacology. 2007;**7**(6):648-652

[72] Lopresti AL, Drummond PD. Obesity and psychiatric disorders: Commonalities in dysregulated biological pathways and their implications for treatment. Progress in Neuro-Psychopharmacology & Biological Psychiatry. 2013;**45**:92-99

[73] Quek YH, Tam WW, Zhang MW, Ho R. Exploring the association between childhood and adolescent obesity and depression: A meta-analysis. Obesity Reviews. 2017;**18**(7):742-754

[74] Mannan M, Mamun A, Doi S, Clavarino A. Prospective associations between depression and obesity for adolescent males and females-a systematic review and meta-analysis of longitudinal studies. PLoS One. 2016;**11**(6):e0157240

[75] Marmorstein NR, Iacono WG, Legrand L. Obesity and depression in adolescence and beyond: Reciprocal risks. International Journal of Obesity. 2014;**38**(7):906-911

[76] Zeller MH, Reiter-Purtill J, Jenkins TM, Ratcliff MB. Adolescent suicidal behavior across the excess weight status spectrum. Obesity. 2013;**21**(5):1039-1045

[77] van Dam RM, Willett WC, Manson JE, Hu FB. The relationship between overweight in adolescence and premature death in women. Annals of Internal Medicine. 2006;**145**(2):91-97

[78] McElroy SL, Kotwal R, Malhotra S, Nelson EB, Keck PE, Nemero CB. Are mood disorders and obesity related? A review for the mental health professional. The Journal of Clinical Psychiatry. 2004;**65**:634-651

[79] McElroy SL, Keck PEJ. Obesity in bipolar disorder: An overview. Current Psychiatry Reports. 2012;**14**:650-658

[80] Goldstein BI, Birmaher B, Axelson DA, Goldstein TR, Esposito-Smythers C, Strober MA, et al. Preliminary findings regarding overweight and obesity in pediatric bipolar disorder. The Journal of Clinical Psychiatry. 2008;**69**:1953-1959

[81] Perugi G, Fornaro M, Akiskal HS. Are atypical depression, borderline personality disorder and bipolar II disorder overlapping manifestations of a common cyclothymic diathesis? World Psychiatry. 2011;**10**:45-51

[82] Perugi G, Akiskal HS, Lattanzi L, Cecconi D, Mastrocinque C, Patronelli A, et al. The high prevalence of "soft" bipolar (II) features in atypical depression. Comprehensive Psychiatry. 1998;**39**:63-71

[83] Calkin C, Van De Velde C, Růžičková M, Slaney C, Garnham J, Hajek T, et al. Can body mass index help predict outcome in patients with bipolar disorder? Bipolar Disorders. 2009;**11**(6):650-656

[84] McElroy SL, Kemp DE, Friedman ES, Reilly-Harrington NA, Sylvia LG, Calabrese JR, et al. Obesity, but not metabolic syndrome, negatively

affects outcome in bipolar disorder. Acta Psychiatrica Scandinavica. 2016;**133**(2):144-153

[85] Shapiro J, Mindra S, Timmins V, Swampillai B, Scavone A, Collinger K, et al. Controlled study of obesity among adolescents with bipolar disorder. Journal of Child and Adolescent Psychopharmacology. 2017;**27**(1):95-100

[86] da Luz FQ, Hay P, Touyz S, Sainsbury A. Obesity with comorbid eating disorders: Associated health risks and treatment approaches. Nutrients. 2018;**10**:829

[87] Segura-Garcia C, Caroleo M, Rania M, Barbuto E, Sinopoli F, Aloi M, et al. Binge eating disorder and bipolar Spectrum disorders in obesity: Psychopathological and eating behaviors differences according to comorbidities. Journal of Affective Disorders. 2017;**208**:424-430

[88] Fornaro M, Perugi G, Gabrielli F, Prestia D, Mattei C, Vinciguerra V, et al. Lifetime co-morbidity with different subtypes of eating disorders in 148 females with bipolar disorders. Journal of Affective Disorders. 2010;**121**:147-151

[89] Villarejo C, Fernández-Aranda F, Jiménez-Murcia S, Peñas-Lledó E, Granero R, Penelo E, et al. Lifetime obesity in patients with eating disorders: Increasing prevalence, clinical and personality correlates. European Eating Disorders Review. 2012;**20**:250-254

[90] Farr OM, Li C-SR, Mantzoros CS. Central nervous system regulation of eating: Insights from human brain imaging. Metabolism. 2016;**65**:699-713

[91] Könner AC, Brüning JC. Selective insulin and leptin resistance in metabolic disorders. Cell Metabolism. 2012;**16**:144-152

[92] Hayes JF, Fitzsimmons-Craft EE, Karam AM, Jakubiak J, Brown ML, Wilfley DE. Disordered eating attitudes and behaviors in youth with overweight and obesity: Implications for treatment. Current Obesity Reports. 2018;**7**:235-246

[93] De Velasco RM, Barbudo E, Pérez-Templado J, Silveira B, Quintero J. Review of the association between obesity and ADHD. Actas Españolas de Psiquiatría. 2015;**43**:16-23

[94] Ziauddeen H, Alonso-Alonso M, Hill JO, Kelley M, Khan NA. Obesity and the neurocognitive basis of food reward and the control of intake. Advances in Nutrition. 2015;**6**:474-486

[95] McCuen-Wurst C, Ruggieri M, Allison KC. Disordered eating and obesity: Associations between binge-eating disorder, night-eating syndrome, and weight-related comorbidities. Annals of the New York Academy of Sciences. 2018;**1411**:96-10

[96] Blum K, Thanos PK, Gold MS. Dopamine and glucose, obesity and reward deficiency syndrome. Frontiers in Psychology. 2014;**5**:1-11

[97] Jebb SA, Prentice AM. Is obesity an eating disorder? The Proceedings of the Nutrition Society. 1995;**54**:721-728

[98] Jemma DAY, Ternouth A, Collier DA. Eating disorders and obesity: Two sides of the same coin? Epidemiologia e Psichiatria Sociale. 2009;**18**:96-100

[99] Raman J, Smith E, Hay P. The clinical obesity maintenance model: An integration of psychological constructs including mood, emotional regulation, disordered overeating, habitual cluster behaviours, health literacy and cognitive function. Journal of Obesity. 2013;**2013**:240128

[100] Dingemans A, Danner U, Parks M. Emotion regulation in binge eating disorder: A review. Nutrients. 2017;**9**:1274

[101] Van Strien T. Causes of emotional eating and matched treatment of obesity. Current Diabetes Reports. 2018;**18**:35

[102] Raevuori A, Suokas J, Haukka J, Gissler M, Linna M, Grainger M, et al. Highly increased risk of type 2 diabetes in patients with binge eating disorder and bulimia nervosa. The International Journal of Eating Disorders. 2015;**48**:555-562

[103] Succurro E, Segura-Garcia C, Ruo M, Caroleo M, Rania M, Aloi M, et al. Obese patients with a binge eating disorder have an unfavorable metabolic and inflammatory profile. Medicine. 2015;**94**:e2098

[104] Zhang J, Abbasi O, Malevanchik L, Mohan N, Denicola R, Tarangelo N, et al. Pilot study of the prevalence of binge eating disorder in non-alcoholic fatty liver disease patients. Annals of Gastroenterology. 2017;**30**:664-669

[105] Wassenaar E, Friedman J, Mehler PS. Medical complications of binge eating disorder. Psychiatric Clinics of North America. 2019;**42**:275-286

[106] Kessler RC, Berglund PA, Chiu WT, Deitz AC, Hudson JI, Shahly V, et al. The prevalence and correlates of binge eating disorder in the World Health Organization world mental health surveys. Biological Psychiatry. 2013;**73**:904-914

[107] Cortese S, Moreira-Maia CR, St Fleur D, Morcillo-Peñalver C, Rohde LA, Faraone SV. Association between ADHD and obesity: A systematic review and meta-analysis. The American Journal of Psychiatry. 2016;**173**:34-43

[108] Sönmez AÖ, Yavuz BG, Aka S, Semiz S. Attention-deficit hyperactivity disorder symptoms and conduct problems in children and adolescents with obesity. The Medical Bulletin of SISLI ETFAL Hospital. 2019;**53**:300-305

[109] Martins-Silva T, Vaz JDS, Hutz MH, Salatino-Oliveira A, Genro JP, Hartwig FP, et al. Assessing causality in the association between attention-deficit/hyperactivity disorder and obesity: A Mendelian randomization study. International Journal of Obesity. 2019;**43**:2500-2508

[110] Seymour KE, Reinblatt SP, Benson L, Carnell S, Sciences B. Overlapping neurobehavioral circuits in ADHD, obesity, and binge eating: Evidence from neuroimaging research. CNS Spectrums. 2016;**20**:401-411

[111] VanVeen MM, Kooij JJS, Boonstra AM, Gordijn MCM, Van Someren EJW. Delayed circadian rhythm in adults with attention-deficit/hyperactivity disorder and chronic sleep-onset insomnia. Biological Psychiatry. 2010;**67**:1091-1096

[112] Vogel SWN, Bijlenga D, Tanke M, Bron TI, van der Heijden KB, Swaab H, et al. Circadian rhythm disruption as a link between attention-deficit/hyperactivity disorder and obesity? Journal of Psychosomatic Research. 2015;**79**:443-450

[113] Verbeken S, Braet C, Goossens L, van der Oord S. Executive function training with game elements for obese children: A novel treatment to enhance self-regulatory abilities for weight-control. Behaviour Research and Therapy. 2013;**51**:290-299. Available from: https://www.cdc.gov/obesity/strategies/obesity-strategies-what-can-be-done.html

Section 2

New Perspectives in Obesity Management and Treatment

Chapter 3

Treatment of Adults with Obesity Using the Unified Health System: An Interdisciplinary Proposal

Liz Elaine Sowek, Marcia Regina Carletto and Erildo Vicente Muller

Abstract

Obesity is a multifactorial chronic disease requiring interdisciplinary care. This study aimed to evaluate the impact of a group-based interdisciplinary intervention for adults with obesity using the Unified Health System (SUS). Conducted in Ponta Grossa, PR, from October 2018 to June 2019, qualitative data were gathered through semi-structured interviews with nine participants selected based on significant quantitative outcomes. A clinical and sociodemographic questionnaire supported the data collection. Data were analyzed using Bardin's content analysis and QDAS Nvivo 11 software. The intervention emphasized cognitive restructuring, self-monitoring, gamification, coping strategies, and nutritional education, led by a dietitian, psychologist, and physical educator. Participants reported improvements in self-awareness, behavioral changes, and health literacy. Key themes included enhanced emotional regulation, motivation for lifestyle modifications, and perceived benefits of group dynamics. These findings underscore the potential for replicating low-cost, interdisciplinary interventions in public health systems, offering substantial psychosocial and behavioral benefits in managing obesity.

Keywords: obesity, interdisciplinary intervention, qualitative analysis, behavioral change, public health

1. Introduction

Chronic non-communicable diseases (NCDs) represent a significant challenge to global public health due to their complexity and difficulty in control, requiring a healthcare model that incorporates health promotion, prevention, and treatment strategies [1]. Obesity, a chronic and multifactorial disease with epigenetic interactions, is a major risk factor for comorbidities such as diabetes mellitus, dyslipidemia, hypertension, cardiovascular diseases, certain cancers, non-alcoholic fatty liver disease, asthma, sleep disorders, mood disorders, and eating disorders [2, 3].

Historically, obesity has been recognized since ancient times, with early anti-obesity recommendations focusing on diet, exercise, and lifestyle changes [4]. Today, obesity has become a global epidemic, imposing a significant burden on society and public health systems due to its association with high morbidity and mortality [5]. Worldwide, it is estimated that by 2025, approximately 2.3 billion adults will be overweight, and over 700 million will be obese. In Brazil, the prevalence of obesity has increased by 67.8% (from 11.8% in 2006 to 19.8% in 2018), highlighting the urgent need for organized healthcare services to address this growing demand [6].

Prevention and control of obesity require integrated actions that support individuals in adopting healthy lifestyles and maintaining or achieving a healthy weight. Health Care Networks (RAS) play a crucial role in optimizing care at micro (individuals and families), meso (health services and communities), and macro (health policies) levels, promoting intersectoral collaboration and interdisciplinary approaches [7, 8]. However, traditional unidisciplinary treatments often result in temporary weight loss, underscoring the need for interdisciplinary strategies that address the multifactorial nature of obesity and promote sustainable behavioral changes [1, 9].

The interest in researching this topic arose from my professional trajectory, where I identified a gap in obesity treatment within primary care. My academic background in nutrition and work as a nutritionist in the Family Health Support Center (NASF) significantly influenced this research. The simplistic approach of some professionals led me to recognize that obesity care was often individualized, fragmented, costly, and low in resoluteness. This highlighted the need for partnerships to address such a complex and multifactorial disease, as treating obesity unidimensionally would be like "blowing a fan at the tip of an iceberg and expecting it to change direction." Therefore, I sought to develop and implement an interdisciplinary proposal for the treatment of adults with obesity using the Brazilian Unified Health System (SUS).

This chapter focuses exclusively on the qualitative findings of a study that implemented an interdisciplinary group intervention for adults with obesity using the Brazilian Unified Health System (SUS). The intervention, conducted in Ponta Grossa-PR between October 2018 and June 2019, involved nutritionists, psychologists, and physical educators using techniques such as cognitive restructuring, self-monitoring, gamification, and nutritional education. The qualitative analysis aimed to explore participants' experiences, perceptions, and behavioral changes, providing insights into the psychosocial dimensions of obesity treatment. By presenting these findings, this chapter contributes to the development of low-cost, interdisciplinary models for obesity care in public health systems.

2. Materials and methods

2.1 Study type

It is classified as a quasi-experimental, non-controlled, mixed-methods study, comparing different indicators of subjects who participated in an interdisciplinary group intervention at two distinct moments: baseline and a follow-up 8 weeks after the end of each group.

2.2 Sample definition

The sample was intentionally selected (convenience sampling) due to the need for an intervention focused on Brazilian Unified Health System (SUS) users diagnosed with obesity, experiencing the consequences of the disease, and willing to participate in the research.

2.3 Research stages

The research was developed in two stages: the first, quantitative, and the second, qualitative, both with three phases each. The qualitative stage was conducted after the intervention, following three steps: (1) interviews with the four participants from each group who showed the best results, (2) transcription and validation, and (3) data analysis.

2.4 Ethical considerations

In accordance with the Guidelines and Regulatory Standards for research involving human subjects, as established by Resolution CNS No. 466/2012, this study was submitted to the Research Ethics Committee of the State University of Ponta Grossa and approved under opinion No. 2.910.450.

2.5 Semi-structured interview

This instrument was chosen because it allows greater interaction between the interviewee and the interviewer, facilitating clarification and deeper exploration of issues related to the research interests. The interview was developed by the author and consists of 14 questions divided into three domains (behavioral, health, and post-intervention outcomes), addressing topics such as habit changes, self-esteem, and physical activity.

2.6 Participants and research location

The study participants were users of primary healthcare units who were identified as needing habit and behavior changes. They were referred by physicians, nurses, and community health agents, while some learned about the project through various media channels promoted by the Communication Department of the Municipal Government.

The research was conducted between October 2018 and July 2019 in the city of Ponta Grossa, Paraná, Brazil. Each group was initially composed of 33 individuals, a number determined by the physical space limitations and considering a potential sample loss of 50%, ensuring a still significant sample size. The first group concluded with 16 participants, the second with 17, and the third with 11. Ultimately, due to various reasons, the average number of participants who completed the sessions was 44% of those initially selected. Dropouts occurred due to absences exceeding two meetings, conflicts with the scheduled days and times, travel, new job opportunities, and failure to complete the required laboratory tests.

2.7 Research procedures

1. First moment of the first stage—initial questionnaire was applied, and anthropometric and biochemical parameters were collected.

2. Second moment of the first stage—the intervention.

Three groups were formed at different periods, each participating in nine weekly sessions lasting approximately two and a half hours. The intervention was named

"New Shape" ("Nova Forma"). Three professionals facilitated the sessions: a nutritionist (the study researcher), a psychologist, and a physical educator. Additionally, nutrition interns and public health residents (pharmacists, nutritionists, physiotherapists, and veterinary doctors) participated in the intervention. The nutritionist, residents, and interns attended all sessions, while the psychologist participated in three sessions and the physical educator in five.

The main techniques used during the meetings were cognitive restructuring, self-monitoring, gamification, coping card, and nutritional education.

2.7.1 First and second moment: Post-intervention

At this stage, a qualitative analysis was conducted, and the target audience consisted of four participants from each group who showed significant results in the quantitative analysis. Characterized as a purposive sample, this group underwent a semi-structured interview, which was recorded and later transcribed with the participants' consent.

Of the total of 12 participants selected for this stage, 9 took part in the interview—all of them women—resulting in a 25% sample loss. The first group had four participants, while the second had 3, as one participant was unable to attend the interview. In the third and final group, three people agreed to participate in the interview, but one of them (the one with the best result) was excluded from the study for not having undergone the required laboratory tests, despite multiple requests.

To validate the interviews, the transcriptions were sent *via* email or delivered in person to each interviewee. They were given the opportunity to read, confirm their statements, and modify their responses if they deemed it necessary. At the end of this process, all participants agreed with the transcriptions, ensuring the validity of the collected data.

3. Data analysis

3.1 Qualitative analysis

The qualitative analysis was conducted using content analysis as proposed by Bardin [10]. This method works with words and allows for a practical and objective understanding of what lies behind the discourses. That is, content analysis is a set of techniques aimed at producing inferences from the content of communication in a text, which can be replicable within its social context. In the analysis, the text is a means of expression by the subject, where the analyst seeks to categorize recurring units of text (words or phrases), inferring an expression that represents them. It is a fast and effective technique when applied to direct and simple discourses [11].

For each interview question, the content analysis was conducted following the three phases proposed by Bardin [10]: (I) pre-analysis, in which, based on the "floating reading" of the texts, initial ideas were organized and systematized, resulting in an analysis plan; (II) exploration of the material, in which the decisions made were systematically applied, and raw data were categorized; and (III) data processing and interpretation, in which results were inferred and compared with the theoretical framework used.

For the exploration of the material and data processing, the QDAS Nvivo 11 software was used, enabling the calculation of word frequency, construction of word clouds (where the size of the words is proportional to their frequency—larger words are more frequent, and smaller words are less frequent), and, finally, cluster analysis of the themes from question 3 based on the similarity of words and their respective sources. The more clustered the themes are, the more sources they share in common, meaning that the grouped themes are likely repeatedly cited by different individuals.

After the intervention, the analyzed data were classified based on common aspects contained in the information or on the divergent positions that stood out. From these real data, extracted from the testimonies that symbolized the experiences and thought styles of the [12] subjects, the possibility of re-elaborating new, more specific categories emerged, as proposed by Cruz [13]. This adaptation can be better visualized in **Table 1**.

After defining the context units, the recording units were established, as presented in **Table 2**.

A—Priori categories		**B—Posteriori categories**	
A	Starting point—in the reign of consumption, immediate pleasure, and sedentary lifestyle	A	Starting point—in the reign of consumption, immediate pleasure, and sedentary lifestyle
B	Lifestyle changes—primary and secondary gains	B	Lifestyle changes—primary and secondary gains
C	Impact on health and well-being	C	Impact on health and well-being
		D	Support from the team and the group

Source: The Author.

Table 1.
Content analysis: Adaptation of a priori and a posteriori categorization.

Context unit	**Record unit**
Starting point—In the reign of consumption, immediate pleasure, and sedentary lifestyle	A. Mental health
	B. I used to get sick and had abnormal test results.
	C. I felt unwell, tired, unmotivated, and had low self-esteem.
Lifestyle changes—Primary and secondary gains	A. The desire to eat is anxiety.
	B. I modified my menu.
	C. Today I eat more slowly.
	D. I take better care of my family's diet
Impact on health and well-being	A. In diet.
	B. In physical activity.
	C. Yes, I feel much better.
	D. In my appearance and self-esteem.
Support from the team and the group	A. I could not do it alone.

Source: The Author.

Table 2.
Content analysis: Definition of context units with their respective record units.

4. Results and discussion of qualitative data

4.1 Characterization of the qualitative sample

The group of nine interviewees consisted entirely of women, with two aged between 31 and 40 years, three aged between 41 and 50 years, and four aged between 50 and 60 years. All participants reported weight loss during their participation in the group, ranging from 2.8 to 8.0 kg, with an average weight loss of 6.256 kg. In compliance with the commitment made and documented through the Informed Consent Form (ICF), the identity of the participants was protected. For this reason, the participants were assigned fictitious names: Joana, Maria, Priscila, Caroline, Cleusa, Larissa, Talita, Pamela, and Viviane.

4.2 Content and discussion of the discourses

After the documentary analysis and the data obtained through content analysis from the perspective of Bardin, the results obtained will be presented in detail below.

4.2.1 Starting point: In the reign of consumption, immediate pleasure, and sedentary lifestyle

This context unit brought to light the feelings, discomforts, and problems of obese individuals regarding their excess weight, as corroborated by Zottis and Labronici [14], who state that: the obese body, due to low self-esteem, carries a sense of dissatisfaction, a feeling of worthlessness accompanied by self-deprecation and self-reproach—that is, guilt, weakness, rejection, inferiority, and fragility. The recording units presented below emerged from the first question asked to the interviewees, which was about what motivated them to join a weight loss group. This question allowed data to surface regarding feelings of discomfort, physical complaints, and a strong desire for change.

4.2.1.1 Mental health

Among the issues mentioned were numerous failed attempts to lose weight, feelings of frustration, sadness, guilt, depression, and isolation. The data collected showed that 9 (100%) of the interviewees reported how excess weight affected their mental health, as can be seen in the accounts of Joana and Caroline:

> *[...] Leaving the house was a suffering for me. I had reached a point where I thought everyone would notice me, everyone would judge me [...] (Joana)*

> *[...] I prayed a lot to God because I wanted a way, a solution, because I did not know where I was heading anymore. I gained 15 kilograms in 6 months, and my marriage almost ended [...] (Caroline)*

In general, individuals with obesity experience various types of treatments for weight loss, and anything offered to them regarding weight loss is accepted without concern for possible side effects, especially if the treatment is an easy method that does not require significant effort. This fact is confirmed in the statement of Viviane:

[...] I tried many times on my own, like at home, with medication, with all those things. Everything I saw others doing, I did the same, and it did not work. My weight only increased [...] and then I felt really bad (Viviane).

In Joana's testimony, the feeling of low self-esteem and the need for isolation is evident. This statement confirms what Del Priore [15] states: "Anyone who deviates from the 'beauty standard'—formed by white skin, straight hair, light eyes, and a slim, slender body—is susceptible to judgment, rejection, and criticism."

In Caroline's statement, the desire for change is evident. The strong desire for change in individuals with obesity derives from physical pain and pain associated with their body image.

What is clear is that the desire to change or reprogram a specific habit only occurs when there is discomfort and dissatisfaction.

Another issue that emerged from the participants' statements concerns the comorbidities resulting from obesity, giving rise to the second recording unit.

4.2.1.2 I used to get sick and had abnormal test results

The interviewees' statements regarding health issues confirmed the quantitative data, which indicated a prevalence of hypertension in 56.8% (n = 25), followed by dyslipidemia in 18% (n = 8), and diabetes mellitus in 11.4% (n = 5). The development of comorbidities is an inevitable consequence of obesity. Among the interviewees, 2 (22.2%) stated that hypertension was what drove their desire for change, as can be seen in the statements of Priscila and Talita, respectively:

[...] I went for a consultation, and the doctor said I was pre-diabetic and that my blood pressure was very high, usually 21 over 10 [...] (Priscila).

[...] I thought, if I keep eating like this, I'm going to die because my blood pressure will rise even more [...] (Talita).

The statements of Priscila and Talita are corroborated by Galvão [16] and Sacks [17], who state that individuals with obesity have up to three times the risk of developing hypertension (HTN) and that there is a positive relationship between obesity and the prevalence of HTN. Additionally, it can be observed that 1 (11.1%) of the participants are aware of the effects of excesses on their health, as reported below by Pamela:

[...] I used to get headaches. I overdid it with salt, my blood pressure would rise, I overdid it with food, with junk food. I ate everything daily, overdid it with snacks [...] (Pamela).

The risk factors associated with hypertension (HTN) include inadequate diet, excessive salt intake, abusive alcohol consumption, physical inactivity, excess weight, smoking, and disturbances in glucose and lipid metabolism. Maria mentioned how their immunity was affected, stating:

[...] This issue of low immunity, because, my goodness, I do not know how many times I... last year I almost died because I got pneumonia, and from pneumonia, I got a kidney infection[...] (Maria).

Since obesity is considered an inflammatory disease, and a diet rich in simple carbohydrates and fats favors intestinal bacterial imbalance, increases insulin resistance, and affects the body's defense systems, it is understood that obese individuals are aware of the gradual deterioration of their health. They understand that they are depleting their physical resources by committing dietary excesses and abuses. However, they need encouragement, support, and opportunities for change. In this sense, interdisciplinary and interprofessional support emerges as a key factor in helping them overcome discouragement and low self-esteem resulting from the physical and emotional impairment caused by obesity.

4.2.1.3 I felt unwell, tired, discouraged, and had low self-esteem

This recording unit shows how individuals with obesity struggle to perform simple daily tasks, such as household chores and personal hygiene. Routine tasks become a source of suffering, and losing weight means regaining quality of life, autonomy, and self-esteem—that is, resuming daily activities and reintegrating into their social roles.

In the reports of all nine participants (100%), it was found that excess weight is fundamentally connected to the appearance of clinical symptoms and reduced dexterity and motivation for work. Feelings of tiredness, dissatisfaction, low self-esteem, shame, malaise, anxiety, anguish, sadness, and depression are recurrent:

> *[...] Even cleaning my house was difficult. I felt heavy and tired [...] (Talita).*
>
> *[...] I felt so tired, heavy, I did not have the courage to play with my 6-year-old son [...] (Pamela).*
>
> *[...] Everything I felt was bad—fatigue, malaise [...] (Viviane).*
>
> *[...] I was feeling bad. I looked in the mirror and did not feel good about myself. To do my work, my movements, I wasn't feeling well [...] (Cleusa).*
>
> *[...] Depression, discouragement—you do not feel like taking care of yourself, you let yourself go, you stop living, really [...] (Maria).*
>
> *[...] I felt heavy, bloated, tired, unmotivated. I did not feel like dressing up or even buying clothes [...] (Viviane).*
>
> *[...] You know, I stopped changing clothes in front of my husband [...] (Joana).*
>
> *[...] So when you start gaining weight, feeling bad, not even being able to take a shower in peace or file your feet, then you start to think, 'Hey, something has to change' [...] (Caroline).*

Studies by Kasen et al. [18] indicate that women with a BMI of 30 or more have an increased risk of depression, regardless of other risk factors such as age, education, previous depressive symptoms, marital status, chronic illness, low social support, and financial situation. In addition to bearing the weight of their body, obese individuals carry the weight of guilt and responsibility for their obesity.

It is clear that individuals with obesity face difficulties in socializing and making friends, in taking advantage of opportunities, and in participating in group physical activities, leading to increased food consumption. This occurs because society imposes standards of beauty and youth without respecting ethnic and racial differences, promoting a uniform beauty standard that is practically impossible to achieve.

In the illustrative discourses, it became evident how their emotional balance was affected by excess weight, as they felt inferior due to their body image, exacerbating their low self-esteem. These data reinforce the importance of interdisciplinary work in the treatment of obesity and highlight the significance of the psychologist's role in the intervention. Self-awareness, behavioral change, and respect for individuality are essential in the transformation process.

Therefore, the changes that occurred during the sessions emerge as a context unit, which will now be analyzed.

4.2.2 Lifestyle changes: Primary and secondary gains

The weight loss process requires lifestyle changes (Lifestyle Changes—LC) and behavioral habits. Behavioral changes only occur when there are cognitive modifications. It is believed that individuals with obesity have dysfunctional beliefs regarding food and weight, which end up generating feelings of guilt, anxiety, helplessness, sadness, and difficulties in interpersonal relationships.

For behavioral change to occur, Burch [19] states that stages of conscious competence in knowledge are necessary and involved in the process of progress, moving from "incompetence" to the change of competence in a skill. These stages suggest that, first, individuals are unaware of how little they know about their "incompetence," but when they consciously perceive it, they acquire a skill and can use it. Finally, the skill can be employed even without being conscious of the process, that is, when unconscious competence is acquired. The new behavior occurs through its repetition, positive reinforcement, and self-perception about it.

The registration units depicted in the sequence show the process of change of the intervention participants and their respective gains.

4.2.2.1 The desire to eat is anxiety

The act of eating is multifaceted and does not only mean the intake of nutrients but also encompasses a multitude of emotions and feelings. In this sense, countless times, one "eats" symbolically the anguish, nervousness, anxiety, fear, and frustrations of daily life. When some basic needs are not met, such as high stress, few hours of sleep, and food deprivation, emotional eating can also occur.

If we stop to reflect, from a young age, we are taught to eat for emotional reasons, which becomes a habit; emotion becomes the trigger, and the reward is feeling good. If a child eats everything at lunch, they get dessert; if they cry because their parents are away, they get candy. When we become adults, we only change the pretext of the emotions, but the habit is already formed.

Due to the fact that eating habits have been adopted for a long time, people often do not even realize that their choices are unhealthy. In other situations, even if they identify the need to change their eating habits, it can be very difficult due to various factors, such as work routines and the fact that they do not give proper importance to food. On the other hand, some people desire change, but family or peer influences can hinder it, or they may simply become dependent on certain foods, making it almost impossible to change this habit.

Eating should be guided by bodily sensations, such as hunger, appetite, and satiety—that is, eating when hungry and not just because food is available. Thus, the first step toward achieving this change is being able to distinguish emotional hunger from physiological hunger.

In this sense, all nine interviewees (100%) stated that they knew the difference between hunger and the desire to eat. In the statements below, the participants' perception of identifying this feeling is evident, as well as how they used food as a distraction or comfort for anxiety:

> *[...] "Today I can stop and analyze, you know, is this hunger or anxiety? So I can already identify whether it's stomach hunger or 'that' hunger [...]" (Cleusa)*

> *[...] "The desire to eat is because you're anxious, you want to eat because you're anxious, thinking about a situation you haven't resolved, so you want to kill it with anxiety, so the hunger is a lie [...]" (Talita)*

> *[...] "That hunger hits, and it feels like it even hurts your stomach, but I already see that it's anxiety, so I have to do something to distract myself, and it passes [...]" (Viviane)*

> *[...] "It's like, you see things there, and then, it's not that you're hungry, you just feel like eating. I have my jar of candies, my jar of cookies that I make, covered with icing, super colorful, but today I control myself and can tell the difference [...]" (Caroline)*

> *[...] "Today I know how to deal better with my emotions, right? Sometimes I'm sad, but I don't need to go and eat, eat, eat. I'll eat when I really need to [...]" (Maria)*

> *[...] "I go out, take a walk, I leave the house, go outside, tend to my plants, and I feel that it has passed, so it wasn't hunger to eat, it was 'that' desire [...]" (Cleusa)*

> *[...] "When that crazy desire to eat hits, I have to do something to clear my mind, I'll do something useful [...]" (Joana)*

In the statements of Viviane, Cleusa, Joana, and Maria, it became clear that, after identifying the difference between emotional hunger and physiological hunger, they adopted strategies to manage their emotions without resorting to food. These strategies include engaging in activities such as walking, gardening, or doing something productive, which help them cope with anxiety or emotional triggers without eating unnecessarily.

It is evident that, after the intervention, the participants were able to identify emotional triggers and seek alternative options instead of turning to food, which made them feel more secure and confident. Studies indicate that recognizing eating in response to hunger, desire, and satiety signals is inclined toward healthier eating habits [20, 21].

In Pamela's testimony, it is clear how the tool used during the meetings—the hunger and satiety scale—helped her regain food autonomy and trust in her body's signals:

> *[...] "Often, it was eating more out of anxiety, you know, that thing of, 'Is it tasty? I'll eat more.' A compulsive thing. That scale you shared during the meetings helped me understand the difference [...]" (Pamela)*

DOI: http://dx.doi.org/10.5772/intechopen.1009660

It is evident that the act of eating is closely linked to a person's emotions and how they learned to associate food with filling a void, existential pain, or seeking satisfaction to minimize emotions like fear and anxiety. However, the participants' statements demonstrate that this process can be reversed through learning to differentiate between biological hunger and emotional hunger, as 100% of the interviewees reported a better understanding of their body's signals In the next registration unit, the focus shifts to analyzing changes in eating habits and how food has become important in their lives.

4.2.2.2 I modified my menu

Food preferences have a significant influence on health and well-being, not only physically but also emotionally. What we eat can directly influence how we feel, as our cells are formed by nutrients, which are modifiers and modulators of the human body's response, altering its functioning throughout life.

In this registration unit, all nine participants (100%) reported that after the intervention, they made healthier food choices, replaced or reduced the consumption of certain foods, began reading labels, and made better choices. Most importantly, they recognized the importance of food in their lives and understood that habits and tastes are not unchangeable but rather modifiable.

In the accounts of Talita, Maria and Viviane, it is clear how the stimulus control technique was used when they reported planning their supermarket shopping to avoid purchasing unwanted foods. This allowed them to modify a situation that could have led to a loss of control over eating:

> *[...] "You know, I started realizing that I need to plan my shopping, go to the market, and do the shopping myself. I have to do something for myself (...) even processed products, I'm replacing them. It's a pretty radical change [...]" (Talita)*

> *[...] "I try to shop differently now, more fruits and vegetables. I notice and look at other people's carts, and I think, 'Oh my God! I used to do that, right?' Condensed milk? It's been 2 months since I bought any for my house [...]" (Maria)*

> *[...] "It's like, I look around, I walk through the market thinking everything is toxic. It's funny, for those who know, I look at the shelves, read the labels, and make better choices [...]" (Viviane)*

In Joana's statement, it is evident that she developed a taste for greens and now eats them with pleasure rather than obligation. This aligns with the thinking of behavioral psychologist Köster [22], who states that "we can only change bad eating habits by making healthy food enjoyable. If we try healthy foods out of obligation—as something that requires effort—they will never be appetizing."

> *[...] "I didn't like greens, I didn't like them, I ate them because I had to when I was on a diet. Now, greens are the highlight of my plate. Vegetables, greens, I learned to like them. I really miss them when there's no green food for me [...]" (Joana)*

Another point worth highlighting is that, in the participants' accounts, it is clear that access to information gave them the self-sufficiency to make better choices, plan, and prepare meals. Food and nutrition education provides information that can support people in decision-making, increase their power of choice, and enable them to exercise their autonomy in opting for healthier food choices.

Ultimately, as important as what we eat is how we eat—that is, the scenario surrounding food consumption. Eating in a rush, standing up, alone, or with others are important factors that determine which foods will be consumed and, more importantly, in what quantities. From this context, the next category to be analyzed emerges.

4.2.2.3 Today I eat more slowly

One of the most common characteristics observed in our society regarding eating habits is the tendency to rush through meals. The habit of chewing and swallowing food in just a few seconds dates back to the Paleolithic era and is rooted in the goal of protecting food. Unconscious eating is also prevalent, occurring when people eat while simultaneously engaging in other activities—such as using their phones, watching TV, studying, or working on the computer—allowing these activities to compete with mealtime.

In the statements of all nine interviewees (100%), it is evident that the practice of mindful eating and the tools used during the meetings—such as the set table technique, the chocolate meditation, and the food diary—were decisive in the behavioral change process. The accounts of Cleusa, Maria, and Joana exemplify this:

> *[...] "Ah, eating slowly, paying attention to what I'm eating, how I'm eating, savoring the flavor. So, the pace of eating has changed [...]" (Cleusa)*

> *[...] "I didn't set the table and ate standing up, rushing, not chewing properly. I always thought I didn't eat much, but when I wrote in the food diary, I realized I was eating way more than I thought [...]" (Maria)*

> *[...] "With the meditation, I learned to savor the taste, put the utensils down, breathe, and eat slowly. This helped me eat less [...]" (Joana)*

The practice of increasing attention while eating helps recognize satiety: eating without distractions, focusing on the meal, resting utensils on the plate to evaluate taste and flavor, understanding physical signals, and pausing during the meal. For this, it is important to know that it is okay to leave food on the plate when satisfied or when the food does not taste good—and that it's not necessary to stop only when the package or plate is empty. This builds a learning process around choice. Studies by Kristeller and Wolever [23] indicate that more mindful individuals can reduce binge eating in response to emotional stressors.

Chewing also plays an important role in the habit-changing process. When done slowly, hormonal mechanisms are activated, promoting a feeling of satiety. People who eat more slowly tend to have a lower energy intake compared to those who eat quickly. Continuing with the changes observed after the intervention, we now move on to discuss the next registration unit.

4.2.2.4 I take better care of my family's diet

In this registration unit, it is evident that the benefits of education regarding healthy eating can extend to the family environment and other social groups of the participants, spreading the knowledge built during the intervention. Since women are often responsible for purchasing and preparing food, they have a significant influence on the eating habits of the entire family.

Family eating habits are often reproduced in adulthood, and this has broader social consequences than one might imagine. Improving the eating behavior of parents, especially mothers—including weight loss—can also positively impact the family's dietary profile.

This was no different for most of the interviewees, with seven of them (77.77%) reporting that their habit changes positively influenced their families, as seen in the accounts of Joana and Cleusa:

> *[...] "My family is being supportive of me and also changing their lives [...]" (Joana)*

> *[...] "My husband managed to change, not a complete change, right? He wants to have a healthier life, and he also needed to lose weight [...]" (Cleusa)*

According to Tyler and Horner [24], behaviors and lifestyles are learned within the family, and interventions involving the family, focusing on supportive relationships, can motivate and develop skills for changing eating behaviors.

However, two interviewees (22.22%) reported that their habit changes did not influence their spouses, as expressed in the statements of Caroline. A possible explanation for this is that, culturally, men are often seen as strong and invulnerable, leading them to worry less about their health.

> *[...] "My husband doesn't complain. If I make just a salad, rice, and meat, he'll eat it and won't complain. He doesn't ask for anything (...) but what I wanted was for him to cut down on sweets and soda (...) I tell him that, and he says he won't stop having what he likes. That's fine, I don't drink it, but he does [...]" (Caroline)*

It is in this sense that the family stands out with the potential to maintain eating habits or not. It further reinforces that the family can assist the patient with attitudes that serve as an example for them to adopt healthier eating habits. Thus, it is not enough for the family member to give advice to the obese person about what is correct, but they must also get involved in the process, seeking, for example, to accompany them on walks or also modifying their own eating habits. In this aspect, the family constitutes a source of support for promoting changes.

Thus, this analysis allowed us to verify the behavioral changes that occurred after the intervention, where the development of food competencies could be observed, such as planning purchases, healthier choices, reading labels, and differentiating emotional hunger from physiological hunger. The effects on health and well-being that these changes brought about emerged as the next unit of context that we will discuss.

4.2.3 Impact on health and well-being

Excess weight has significant repercussions on health, psychological well-being, longevity, and quality of life. The treatment of obesity must go beyond weight loss, focusing on improving overall health and long-term well-being. The registration units shown in the sequence derive from the question presented to the participants, which resulted in the improvement of their lives after the intervention. In this way, this question allowed the identification of data on lifestyle changes and improvements in quality of life.

4.2.3.1 Diet

The association between the eating habits of an individual or population and their health status is already extensively known. In low- and middle-income countries, there is an increase in the availability and per capita consumption of food products with high energy density and poor nutrients, which contributes significantly to the obesity epidemic.

It is observed that the consumption of processed and ultra-processed foods is relatively high in the diet of overweight adults, contributing to a greater intake of energy, sugars, and unhealthy fats, along with low fiber content. Monteiro and colleagues [25] emphasize that ultra-processed foods contain less than half the dietary fiber, almost six times the number of free sugars, and significantly more sodium and fat.

In the account of Cleusa and Talita, it is possible to see how the consumption of soft drinks, sweets, and other ultra-processed foods was high before the intervention and how they managed to reduce their intake. This type of food has become the foundation of family diets, often replacing fresh or minimally processed foods due to their hyper-palatability, attractiveness, sophisticated packaging, and aggressive marketing campaigns:

> *[...] I no longer feel that need to always have a soft drink with me. Before, when we went shopping, it seemed like we had to get the soft drink first and then the other household necessities, right? Our shopping habits have changed, yes, they have improved in quality by about 50%—more vegetables, more greens, and fruits. I did not have much of a habit of eating fruit before, but today I consume much more. I do not use sugar anymore [...] (Cleusa)*

> *[...] The habit of eating chocolate and sweets—I go to the store, look at the sweets, and think, they used to relieve my anxiety, but they did not help me at all, they only made me gain more weight. So today, I look at them naturally; I managed to give them up. Oh, and cookies—if I bought those filled wafer cookies, I would eat the whole package in five minutes [...] (Talita)*

In Viviane's statement, one can see how she felt addicted to consuming these ultra-processed foods and how taste perception can change with the intake of food products rich in salt, sugar, fat, chemical additives, preservatives, and flavor enhancers. Especially when consumed daily, people become accustomed to them and reject milder-tasting foods, such as fresh and minimally processed foods:

> *[...] I gave up soft drinks, I do not drink juice either, and I have almost completely eliminated sugar. I realized that it is truly addictive. Once you notice, sweets in general are too. Processed canned foods—everything industrialized—I cut them out because of the project, right? It always encouraged us, and now we know what is right and what is not [...] (Viviane)*

For a lifestyle change, modifying eating habits alone will not yield satisfactory results for improving quality of life and weight loss if it is not associated with physical activity. The activities offered during the intervention in this area and their impact will be discussed in the next recording unit.

4.2.3.2 Physical activity

Weight reduction also leads to a decrease in problems such as back pain, leg pain, and knee pain caused by the overload of weight on the joints, optimizing the individual's movement and the practice of physical exercise [1]. During the intervention, several locations and free exercise options were made available, as one of the barriers preventing people from exercising is the high cost and lack of an adequate place.

Additionally, participants were constantly encouraged to gradually increase their daily physical activity and to seek exercise modalities that were enjoyable and compatible with their routines. The importance of the physical educator in the interdisciplinary team is highlighted here.

The duration of each activity varied from 20 to 90 minutes, with an average of 43.5 minutes. The frequency of activities ranged from 2 to 7 times per week, with an average of five times per week. As observed, eight out of the nine interviewees (88.8%) managed to incorporate physical exercise into their routine. The activities cited were highly diverse and chosen according to each individual's preference.

The duration and frequency were sufficient to maintain good health, as, according to Bouchard et al. [26], 150 minutes of moderate-intensity physical activity per week, distributed throughout the week, are necessary to achieve health benefits.

When asked whether physical activity had helped in their transformation process, 7 (77.77%) interviewees reported that it had. The testimonies of Larissa, Joana, Maria, Talita, and Pamela clearly express their perception of the importance of exercise in the weight loss process, improved energy levels, reduced anxiety, and socialization. This fact is supported by Werneck, Bara Filho, and Ribeiro [27], who state that physical exercise is also important for promoting mental health by improving mood and emotional stability and reducing anxiety and depression:

> *[...] Physical exercise is essential. Diet alone, even though I was doing everything correctly, I realized that I was not able to lose weight, I I lost a lot of inches, I was even impressed [...] (Larissa) [...]*

> *[...] After physical activity, we feel more "relaxed," right? More at ease. We feel less rushed because we also become calmer about food [...] (Joana)*

> *[...] I cannot believe I managed to stop being sedentary. My mood improved, and I feel more energetic [...] (Maria)*

> *[...] I love going to dance class. There, I talk, laugh—it's a moment to unwind and take care of myself [...] (Talita)*

> *[...] Wow, I've grown, developed my best side—I have an athletic spirit inside me. I wake up and do what I have to do. The word 'laziness' is no longer in my vocabulary. I can walk every day, and it's such a great feeling. My body feels light [...] (Pamela)*

However, 2 (22.22%) of the interviewees, Cleusa and Caroline, mentioned that changing their eating habits was the most important factor, as only after improving their diet did, they feel more energized to engage in physical activity. It is well known that a healthy diet is the foundation for achieving optimal health, especially when combined with regular exercise. Likewise, improving health and quality of life can be achieved by transitioning from a sedentary lifestyle and, at the same time, by adopting better eating habits.

As previously mentioned, in addition to comorbidities, obesity leads to emotional, marital, and sexual issues. These matters are closely linked to self-esteem and will be discussed in the next section.

4.2.3.3 My appearance and self-esteem

Body image is shaped by what a person sees in the mirror, forming a mental representation of themselves. This body, perceived uniquely through various senses, can be associated with either a positive or negative self-image, often depending on the approval of others to feel aligned with the "esthetic standards" imposed by society.

When asked about their self-esteem before participating in the intervention, 5 (55.5%) stated it was low, 2 (22.2%) rated it as average, and the remaining 2 (22.2%) considered it good. In contrast, after the intervention, 8 (88.88%) of the interviewees reported that their self-esteem was excellent, while 1 (11.11%) said it was good.

These findings support what was discussed in Registration Unit 1, item C ("I felt unmotivated, tired, discouraged, and had low self-esteem"), highlighting how an obese person's dissatisfaction with their body image can impact their self-esteem. Moreover, after the intervention and weight loss, their self-esteem increased, their mood improved, and a sense of pride in their new body emerged.

This is confirmed in the testimonies of Pamela and Cleusa:

> *[...] My self-esteem improved 100%, there's nothing else to say, right? Girl, I love life, life is wonderful, everything is amazing. My mood improved, and these delicious foods that I did not even know existed—I can lose weight and still enjoy eating [...] (Pamela)*

> *[...] I sent some photos to my sisters. Wow, they loved them! They noticed... I sent pictures of me walking around, and they were like, "Oh my God! You look beautiful, you lost a lot of weight, keep it up." It feels so good to see that. I even sent them to my friend in Goiás, and she said, "Oh, girl, send me that pamphlet, that brochure—I need to do this too!" [...] (Cleusa)*

Obese individuals face difficulties in finding fashionable clothing with quality and at affordable prices. This means they do not have the freedom to buy the clothes they want, having to limit themselves to purchasing what fits them, as can be observed in Larissa's testimony:

> *[...] I was finally able to buy new clothes, and I could choose; I did not have to buy just what fit. I've already changed my style a little, started wearing things I never used before. You start to feel beautiful, and everything changes. Others begin to say, "Wow, what a difference!" You become an inspiration for other people as well [...] (Larissa)*

In Viviane's testimony, it is evident how excess weight interfered with her perception of her body image and how this affected her marital life.

> *[...] I did not feel attractive; now my husband looks at me with desire. For my married life, it has been wonderful. We are women, right? [...] (Viviane)*

DOI: http://dx.doi.org/10.5772/intechopen.1009660

When a woman is not satisfied with her body, she cannot feel beautiful or attractive, and she often replaces sexual pleasure with the pleasure of eating, further aggravating the problem. Thus, this analysis allowed us to verify the benefits of the changes that occurred after the intervention, in terms of diet, physical activity, and increased self-esteem.

4.2.4 Support from the team and the group

Group interventions are alternatives that allow the exchange of experiences, where participants share their achievements and challenges. This creates an encouraging environment, fostering a sense of companionship, solidarity, and motivation. In this context, participants' opinions regarding the support of the interdisciplinary team and the importance of the group in this process of change can be observed.

4.2.4.1 I could not do it alone

Being part of a group that brings together people with common goals provides an experience that can create an environment of great therapeutic value. It can help participants overcome barriers caused by feelings of isolation, mainly by offering them the opportunity to receive feedback and positive suggestions from others who are going through the same challenges [28, 29].

All nine interviewees (100%) stated that the group and the interdisciplinary team were fundamental in the process of change. In Larissa's testimony, she emphasizes how the participation of various professionals working together made a difference in the process, reiterating the importance of the interdisciplinary team:

> *[...] It adds more knowledge because you did not just gather us to ask how our week was; you gathered us, made a schedule, gave a lecture, talked to us, and besides you, there was the psychologist, the physical educator, the residents... it's a lot. So, for those who truly want it, they take advantage of everything, even the testimony of a colleague. [...] (Larissa)*

In the statements of Talita, Joana, and Pamela, it is evident that socializing with people who share a common goal makes the process lighter, creating an atmosphere of companionship, mutual support, and motivation, which strengthens group cohesion:

> *[...] Even the testimony of a colleague. Because then you look and say: Wow! You think you are the only one there, alone in the crowd, and suddenly you start seeing (. .) "Wow, there are people in the group much thinner than me," but everyone has their own problem—one has diabetes, another has a knee problem. And you realize it's not easy; it's not a miracle. [...] (Talita)*

> *[...] I think I would not have achieved this alone; I had tried several times before, and the group helped a lot. [...] (Joana)*

> *[...] This group of yours, this process you follow, is better than Facebook, better than just following things on the internet. You cannot miss sessions because you do not want to lose anything. I think the fact that it's in person makes a difference—you see the food, you talk face to face. [...] (Pamela)*

When asked whether the activities developed in the group provided them with the support to continue on their own, eight out of nine participants (88.88%) said yes. The statements of Viviane, Priscila, Maria, and Larissa reveal that they feel motivated and understand that the process continues—that just because the group meetings have ended, it does not mean they will return to old habits:

> *[...] Definitely. I want to follow this for the rest of my life, even after I reach my desired weight. I will keep going, no doubt about it. As they say, obstacles will always come our way, so we have to be prepared to face them. [...] (Viviane)*

> *[...] I ask God never to let me forget anything I've learned because I do not intend to abandon the habits I developed. Otherwise, I'd be going backward, right? So, in my mind, I do not want to stop doing anything I've learned. [...] (Priscila)*

> *[...] Oh, I want to keep this forever. You have to have a focus, right? Since I feel good today, I want to continue feeling good tomorrow. [...] (Maria)*

> *[...] Ah, I feel a lot, very much, a lot to continue always for the rest of my life. It's no use stopping halfway because everything goes back, it's no use, it's forever[...] (Larissa)*

One of the interviewees (11.11%) reported having the "impression that if she had continued in the group, she would have achieved a bit more" (Talita), although the same interviewee stated that she believes she will be able to continue on her own. Out of the total interviewees, 5 (55.55%) mentioned the virtual WhatsApp group, which keeps them in touch, will provide support to continue with the new habits.

These contributions demonstrated the importance of the activities developed during the intervention for the behavioral change of the study participants, the improvement of self-esteem, the abandonment of the diet mentality, intuitive eating with respect to hunger and satiety sensations, the practice of physical activity with pleasure, and the motivation to continue alone.

Among the limitations of this work are the absence of an experimental design with a control group and the lack of follow-up with participants in a follow-up format, which is another point worth highlighting. In future studies, it is recommended that follow-up sessions be conducted to help participants maintain the skills they have acquired.

Another aspect that should be considered in future interventions is the increase in the intervention's workload, lasting more than nine sessions, as studies with a higher number of sessions found results indicating that the duration of the group is directly related to its effects, especially in anthropometric and biochemical parameters.

New studies can also expand the field of research in intervention groups, identifying the difficulties and limitations faced by those who did not achieve significant results, that is, the worst outcomes. Finally, it is emphasized that the importance of this study lies in offering a ready-to-replicate intervention model for the public health network, with significant social impact and low implementation cost.

5. Conclusion

The group intervention proposal and its results demonstrated that the interdisciplinary approach was a key factor in achieving satisfactory outcomes in changing eating behavior. This was evidenced in the exemplary statements, which highlighted the recognition of emotional and physiological hunger, changes in habits, greater autonomy in food choices, and lifestyle modifications, confirming the effectiveness of the intervention.

The treatment of complex diseases, such as obesity, requires comprehensive patient care and, therefore, an interdisciplinary approach. It has been observed that the concept of interdisciplinarity is increasingly accepted, but in practice, some challenges remain, such as the lack of team spirit, difficulty in sharing information, and insufficient communication techniques that foster empathy and bonding. Many professionals are still not fully prepared to deal with the complexity of health problems, particularly in populations facing various emotional, cultural, and socioeconomic vulnerabilities. These difficulties are largely due to the training of health professionals, which is still linked to pedagogical programs and curricula that are mostly focused on a hospital-centered approach, misaligned with public health concepts that consider human beings in their complexity and entirety.

Based on the results and discussions presented in this study, some practical interventions should be encouraged in health education actions within the SUS, such as continuous support for interdisciplinary rather than merely multidisciplinary practices, the training of nutrition professionals with an emphasis on the use of various tools and strategies that can facilitate behavioral change—rejecting the diet mentality and prioritizing a more compassionate approach to nutrition—the support of municipal and state public management for interdisciplinary actions, the organization of discussion groups on obesity within family health teams, and the promotion of collective and public spaces for physical activity.

Author details

Liz Elaine Sowek[1*], Marcia Regina Carletto[2] and Erildo Vicente Muller[3]

1 Health Sciences, Ponta Grossa State University, Paraná, Brazil

2 Scientific and Technological Education, Ponta Grossa State University, Paraná, Brazil

3 Public Health, Ponta Grossa State University, Paraná, Brazil

*Address all correspondence to: lizsowek@gmail.com

References

[1] Brasil. Ministério da Saúde. Secretaria de Atenção à Saúde. Departamento de Atenção Básica. Estratégias para o Cuidado da Pessoa com Doença Crônica: Obesidade. Brasília: Ministério da Saúde; 2014. 212 p

[2] Dâmaso AR, Masquio DCL, Campos RMS, Da S. Obesidade – Guia prático para profissionais da saúde. 1ª ed. São Paulo: Weight Science; 2014

[3] Lean MEJ, Astrup A, Roberts SB. Making progress on the global crisis of obesity and weight management. BMJ. 2018;**361**:k2538

[4] Balke H, Nocito A. A Trip through the History of Obesity. Vol. 102, No. 2. Suiça: Praxis; 2013. pp. 77-83

[5] Mancini MC et al. Tratado de obesidade. 2ª ed. Rio de Janeiro: Guanabara Koogan; 2015

[6] BRASIL. Ministério da Saúde. Secretaria de Vigilância em Saúde. Departamento de Vigilância de Doenças e Agravos não Transmissíveis e Promoção da Saúde. Vigitel Brasil 2018: vigilância de fatores de risco e proteção para doenças crônicas por inquérito telefônico: estimativas sobre frequência e distribuição sociodemográfica de fatores de risco e proteção para doenças crônicas nas capitais dos 26 estados brasileiros e no Distrito Federal em 2019. Brasília: Ministério da Saúde; 2019. 132p.aq5

[7] Mendes EV. Health care networks. Ciência & Saúde Coletiva. 2010;**15**(5):2297

[8] Brasil. Ministério da Saúde. Política Nacional de Educação Popular em Saúde no Âmbito do Sistema Único de Saúde—PNEPS-SUS. Brasília: Ministério da Saúde; 2013

[9] Varela AL et al. Programa de emagrecimento para mulheres obesas envolvendo variáveis nutricionais, psicológicas e exercício físico. Revista Brasileira de Obesidade, Nutrição e Emagrecimento. 2007;**1**(6):12-27

[10] Bardin L. Análise de conteúdo. Lisboa: Editora Edições 70; 1977

[11] Bardin L. Análise de conteúdo. São Paulo: Edições 70; 2011

[12] Fleck L et al. La Génesis y el Desarrollo de un Hecho Científico: Introducción a la Teoría del Estilo de Pensamiento y del Colectivo de Pensamiento. Madrid: Alianza; 1986

[13] Cruz ON. O trabalho de campo como descoberta e criação. In: Minayo MCS, Organizadora. Pesquisa Social: Teoria, Método e Criatividade. 23rd ed. Petrópolis, RJ: Editora Vozes; 1994

[14] Zottis C, Labronici LM. O corpo obeso e a percepção de si. Cogitare Enfermagem. 2002;**7**(2):21-29

[15] Del Priore M. Corpo a corpo com as mulheres: As transformações do corpo feminino no Brasil. In: Strey MN, Cabeda STL, editors. Corpos e Subjetividades em Exercício Interdisciplinar. Porto Alegre: Edipucrs; 2004. p. 108

[16] Galvão CM, Sawada NO, Rossi LA. A prática baseada em evidências: Considerações teóricas para sua implementação na enfermagem perioperatória. Revista Latino-Americana de Enfermagem. 2002;**10**(5):690-695

[17] Sacks FM et al. Comparison of weight-loss diets with different compositions of fat, protein, and

carbohydrates. The New England Journal of Medicine. 2009;**360**(9):859-873

[18] Kasen S, Cohen P, Chen H, Must A. Obesity and psychopathology in women: A three-decade prospective study. International Journal of Obesity. 2008;**32**(3):558-566

[19] Burch N. Four Stages for Learning any New Skill or Four Stages of Competence Were Developed by Burch while Working at Gordon Training International in the 1970s. CA: Gordon Training International; 1970

[20] Carbonneau E, Roy M, Lamarche B, Provencher V, Bégin C, Robitaille J, et al. A Health at Every Size intervention improves intuitive eating and diet quality in Canadian women. Clinical Nutrition. 2017;**36**(3):747-754

[21] Wooley SC, Garner DM. Obesity treatment: The high cost of false hope. Journal of the American Dietetic Association. 1991;**91**(10):1248-1251

[22] Köster EP. Diversity in the determinants of food choice: A psychological perspective. Food Quality and Preference. 2009;**20**(2):70-82

[23] Kristeller J, Wolever RQ, Sheets V. Mindfulness-based eating awareness training (MB-EAT) for binge eating: A randomized clinical trial. Mindfulness. 2014;**5**:282-297

[24] Tyler DO, Horner SD. Family-centered collaborative negotiation: A model for facilitating behavior change in primary care. Journal of the American Academy of Nurse Practitioners. 2008;**20**(4):194-203

[25] Monteiro CA, Cannon G, Levy RB, Claro RM, Moubarac JC, Martins AP, et al. A new classification of foods based on the extent and purpose of their processing. Public Health Nutrition. 2010;**26**(11):2039-2049

[26] Bouchard C, Blair SN, Haskell WL. Physical Activity and Health. Champaign: Human; 2007

[27] Werneck FZ, Bara Filho MG, Ribeiro LCS. Mecanismos de melhoria do humor após o exercício: Revisitando a hipótese das endorfinas. Revista Brasileira de Ciência e Movimento. 2008;**13**(2):135-144

[28] Silva ALAC, Santos I, Oliveira SR, Figueiredo NMA. Atividades grupais em saúde coletiva: Características, possibilidades e limites. Revista Enfermagem UERJ. 2003;**11**(1):18-24

[29] Munari DB, Lucchese R Medeiros M. Reflexões sobre o uso de atividades grupais na atenção a portadores de doenças crônicas. Cienc Cuid Saude. 2009;**8**(1):148-154

Chapter 4

Strategies for Aerobic and Strength Training Prescription to Optimize Adherence in Overweight and Obese Individuals

Carlos Eduardo Rosa da Silva, Diego Santiago, Eduardo Barbosa, Antonio Roberto Doro, Adriano Verame, Leonardo Lima, Gustavo Almeida, Wilian Santana and Aylton Figueira Jr

Abstract

Physical inactivity is one of the main risk factors for premature mortality, accounting for approximately 2 million deaths annually and having a significant impact on public health. Overweight and obese individuals face even greater challenges in maintaining physical exercise, with high dropout rates and difficulties in losing and maintaining body weight. Although traditional guidelines recommend specific amounts of physical activity, long-term adherence remains a critical issue. Recent research suggests that training prescriptions should consider not only physiological aspects but also the practitioner's affective and motivational responses. This chapter reviews the literature on aerobic and strength training prescription strategies to optimize adherence in overweight and obese individuals. The dual-process, hedonic, and self-determination theories are discussed, highlighting the role of automatic and controlled affective reactions in the formation of exercise habits. Evidence indicates that self-selected intensity, affective valence-based prescription, and social support are effective strategies for increasing adherence. Studies show that individualizing training and considering practitioners' preferences contribute to greater pleasure perception and reduced dropout rates. The integration of these principles into exercise prescription can lead to greater engagement and long-term sustainability. The tripartite prescription model, which combines safety, efficacy, and pleasure, may be a more efficient alternative to promoting continuous physical activity and reducing inactivity among overweight and obese individuals. Therefore, strategies that consider not only intensity and workload but also the subjective exercise experience are essential to transforming exercise into an enjoyable and sustainable practice.

Keywords: exercise adherence, aerobic training, strength training, motivation, hedonic theory, overweight, obesity

1. Introduction

Physical inactivity is directly linked to approximately 2 million deaths per year and is responsible for a decline in overall physical health. It accounts for twice as many deaths as obesity and contributes to an increased risk of premature mortality from all causes [1, 2].

Although the figures regarding overweight and obesity are alarming, the reality of weight loss and maintenance is even more complex. When considering the likelihood of an overweight or obese individual returning to a normal weight, the data is not very encouraging.

A comprehensive study involving approximately 170,000 participants revealed that the likelihood of reducing 5% of body weight or achieving a normal weight is quite low. For men, the probability is only 1 in 1290, while for women, it is 1 in 677. Even when individuals manage to lose weight or reach their desired weight, about 52% regain it [3].

This difficulty can be explained by the Theory of Effort Minimization. According to this theory, the human body tends to avoid any unnecessary effort or excessive energy expenditure. Historically, the reduction in food scarcity and the decrease in energy expenditure have led to energy accumulation, resulting in overweight or obesity. When individuals undergo energy restriction, most end up regaining the lost weight due to a biological response aimed at restoring energy balance [4].

Furthermore, a comparative study on weight loss strategies revealed that severe caloric restriction leads to greater weight loss in the first 6 months. However, weight regain after 3 years causes many individuals to return to nearly their initial weight. Among the available strategies, the combination of physical exercise and a hypocaloric diet stands out as the most effective approach for sustainable weight loss, excluding pharmacological options [5].

According to a recent consensus from the American College of Sports Medicine (ACSM), approximately 150 minutes of moderate-to-vigorous physical activity per week is recommended. For weight loss, the recommendation increases to 200–300 minutes per week at a similar intensity. Over a period of 8–12 weeks, such activity levels can result in a weight loss ranging from 0.5 to 3 kg [6].

Effective strategies for weight loss and maintenance are not limited to physical activity alone. They include the combination of caloric restriction with exercise, such as aerobic training, strength training, mind-body activities like yoga, and balance exercises. When these strategies are combined with a negative energy balance, they lead to significant improvements in body composition. This includes reductions in adiposity and visceral fat, as well as enhancements in muscle function, cardiorespiratory capacity, muscle strength, balance, and movement quality.

These factors not only contribute to better body composition but also improve overall health and quality of life. However, adherence to these habits can be challenging. Many individuals struggle to consistently follow these recommendations and maintain an active and healthy lifestyle.

2. Literature review

A recent systematic review analyzed adherence to aerobic and strength training guidelines across more than 31 countries, involving over 3 million participants. The results showed that only 17.15% of adults over the age of 18 follow both guidelines.

Among adolescents aged 12–17, this number increases slightly to 19.45%. This means that, on average, only 1 in 5 adolescents and adults manage to meet the recommended levels of combined aerobic and strength exercise [7].

A study evaluated the dropout rate among gym members, monitoring 5240 individuals over 12 months or until they discontinued their activities. The results showed that the likelihood of dropping out before the third month was 63%. After 12 months, fewer than 4% of those who started the exercise program continued practicing [8].

In 1982, Rod Dishman challenged physical education professionals to find a balance between the ideal physiological prescription and a behavioral prescription that is both feasible and appealing to individuals. Although significant progress has been made in understanding the exercise doses that generate positive adaptations in various body systems, an important gap remains: we still do not know exactly what dose of exercise truly encourages adherence and the long-term maintenance of exercise programs [9].

The greatest challenge for exercise science, therefore, is not only to create effective programs that promote biological adaptations but also to offer training options that individuals willingly adopt on a regular basis throughout their lives [10].

To this day, it seems that we have not yet identified the "ideal dose" that encourages participants to remain engaged over long periods. When considering physical exercise, our brain operates with two types of precursors. Automatic precursors are instinctive affective reactions that make us want to approach or avoid a given activity, while controlled precursors involve more rational attitudes and conscious intentions. These two precursors, along with moderators such as habits, cognition, and mood, determine whether or not we will engage in a health-related behavior, as shown in **Figure 1**.

This idea is part of the dual-process theory, which helps to understand how to predict the long-term maintenance of health and exercise-related behaviors. In other words, slogans like "no pain, no gain" do not seem to be the best approach to attract overweight individuals or those with low physical fitness to engage in regular physical exercise. The dual-process theory suggests that automatic affective reactions, such as the perception of pleasure or displeasure during exercise, are the strongest predictors of maintaining exercise-related behavior.

Structure of the dual-process model for predicting health-related behaviors.

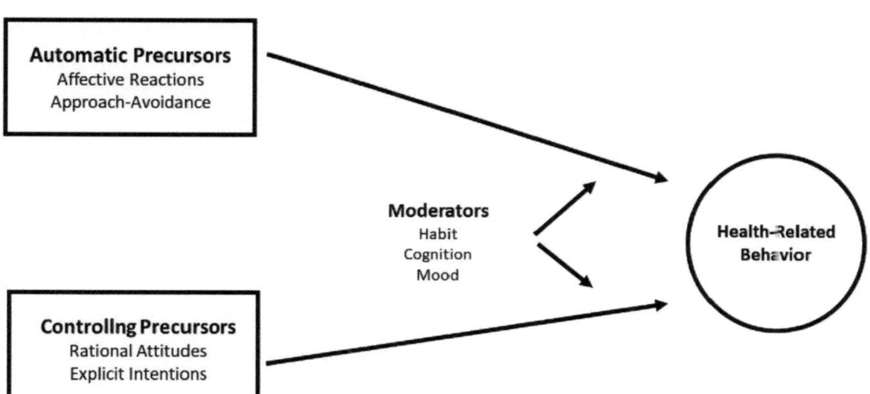

Figure 1.
"Dual process model for health behavior" adapted from Ref. [4].

2.1 Automatic precursors

- Affective reactions: Emotional responses that influence the decision to approach or avoid health-related behaviors.
- Approach-avoidance: Instinctive tendencies that lead an individual to engage in or withdraw from healthy activities.

2.2 Moderators

- Factors influencing the relationship between precursors and behavior:
- Habituality: The influence of established habits on health choices.
- Cognitive load: The impact of available mental capacity on decision-making.
- Mood: How emotional state affects motivation to engage in healthy activities.

2.3 Controlled precursors

- Rational attitudes: Thoughtful evaluations of the benefits and drawbacks of engaging in health behaviors.
- Explicit intentions: Conscious commitments to performing activities that promote health.

2.4 Health-related behavior

The intersection of automatic and controlled precursors, mediated by moderators, results in decisions regarding the adoption and maintenance of healthy habits.

Physical education professionals often prescribe training using a bipartite model, which focuses on the effectiveness and safety of exercise programs. However, some authors suggest expanding this concept into a tripartite model that, in addition to effectiveness and safety, also considers pleasure and the sense of well-being during exercise. The perception of pleasure is a crucial factor, as it is directly linked to the intention to repeat exercise sessions and to the long-term maintenance of exercise-related behavior [11].

Affective responses to physical exercise can be either automatic or cognitive and occur before, during, or after the activity. These variations in effect may be associated with future behavior, influencing whether an individual will continue with a training program. When exercise is perceived as enjoyable, there is a greater potential for long-term adherence and continuity of practice [12, 13].

In a study with 250 gym members followed over 1 year, it was found that only 37% maintained regular exercise practice, training at least twice a week after 1 year. Among those who continued the program, the perception of pleasure, the sense of effort, and the challenge of goal-setting were the main factors associated with greater participation in regular exercise. This reinforces the importance of creating positive experiences during exercise sessions to promote long-term engagement [14].

The dual-mode theory suggests that aerobic exercise at moderate intensities provides a homogeneous response zone where most individuals experience a greater perception of pleasure. This physiological zone is located just below the first ventilatory threshold. As exercise intensity increases, between the first ventilatory threshold and the respiratory compensation point, individuals enter a vigorous intensity zone, in which some begin to experience displeasure, while others still maintain a sense of pleasure. This response zone varies from person to person [13].

When surpassing the respiratory compensation point and approaching VO2 peak, the perception becomes more homogeneous, with most individuals experiencing displeasure. Specifically, in the severe exercise zone, above the respiratory compensation point and close to VO2 peak, discomfort is almost universal (**Figure 2**) [13].

This response pattern is particularly relevant for individuals who are physically inactive, overweight or obese, and have low fitness levels, as they often experience displeasure even during light activities such as walking for transportation, cycling at a slow pace, playing with children, or washing a car. For these individuals, it is essential to identify physical activity options that are not only effective and safe but also provide pleasure and a sense of well-being. This may be the key to promoting long-term adherence and improving quality of life.

A study with 485 participants investigated the discrepancy between intensity preferences and prescribed intensity in physical training, evaluating its impact on perceived vitality, habit formation, and weekly exercise frequency. The results showed that the preferred intensity for most participants was moderate. When the prescribed intensity aligned with the preferred intensity, participants reported higher vitality scores, established more consistent habits, and had a higher exercise frequency [16].

These findings suggest that prescribing training intensities that do not align with individual preferences may risk compromising adherence to training in the medium and long term. Therefore, considering personal preferences when adjusting exercise intensity can be an important strategy to promote engagement and the long-term maintenance of regular physical activity.

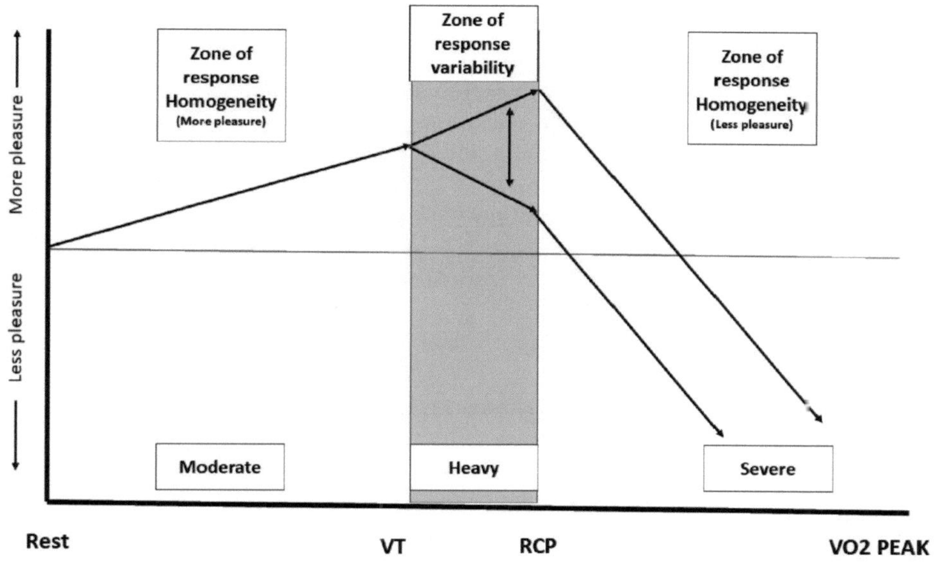

Figure 2.
Representation of the dual-mode theory for continuous exercise at intensities below, at, and above the ventilatory threshold. Ventilatory threshold (VT), Respiratory compensation point (RCP), and Peak oxygen consumption (VO2 peak) [13, 15].

The Self-Determination Theory suggests that the improvement of behavioral regulations related to motivation for physical exercise is directly linked to the fulfillment of basic psychological needs: autonomy, competence, and relatedness. When training is prescribed with adequate support for these needs, individuals are more likely to develop higher-quality motivation, characterized by more self-determined and sustainable behavior [17].

Similarly, the Hedonic Theory suggests that people tend to repeat behaviors they perceive as pleasurable and avoid those that cause discomfort. Positive experiences during exercise are essential for promoting adherence and the continuity of training programs [18].

3. Discussion

Therefore, by combining these two approaches, we can develop strategies that not only fulfill basic psychological needs but also make physical exercise a more enjoyable experience. This may be key to keeping individuals engaged in exercise programs in the medium and long term, promoting not only health but also psychological well-being.

We can apply the concepts of hedonic theory to exercise prescription. An effective strategy is monitoring the perception of pleasure and displeasure during training sessions. This monitoring can be conducted at the end of a set-in strength training or during aerobic exercise, whether continuous or interval-based. Assessing the perception of pleasure or displeasure provides a clear indication of how an individual feels while performing the exercise, allowing for intensity adjustments that can help promote a positive training experience.

Thus, the Feeling Scale is an instrument used to monitor affective responses (pleasure/displeasure) during exercise sessions. It is an 11-point bipolar scale of central affect, ranging from +5 ("very good") to −5 ("very bad"), used as a measure of pleasure and displeasure (**Figure 3**).

In this context, positive scores (+5 to +1) indicate a perception of pleasure, while negative scores (−1 to −5) reflect a perception of displeasure. The neutral score (0) represents the transition point between pleasure and displeasure. The use of this

How are you feeling now?

+5	**Very Good**
+4	
+3	**Good**
+2	
+1	**Reasonably Good**
0	
-1	**Reasonably Bad**
-2	
-3	**Bad**
-4	
-5	**Very Bad**

Figure 3.
Felling scale [19].

instrument can be anchored by a guiding question: During physical exercise, some individuals may experience pleasure or displeasure. At this exact moment, how are you feeling?

It is important to emphasize that affective valence is based on the exact moment of the action or exercise. In this case, it does not refer to past experiences, previous sessions, or prior exercise practices. This assessment is free of judgment (there is no right or wrong) and reflects the individual's perception at the moment of the exercise.

A proposed exercise prescription based on affect-guided training was studied with more than 47 participants, with outcomes including gym attendance, perception of pleasure during the exercise session, post-session pleasure, and anticipated pleasure regarding the expectation of performing the session again. Participants engaged in aerobic and strength training sessions, comparing traditionally prescribed intensities with those guided by the perception of pleasure. The results showed that the training loads in both approaches—prescribed intensity and affect-guided intensity—were similar in terms of intensity and volume. However, participants who followed the affect-guided intensity reported a greater perception of pleasure during the session, more post-exercise pleasure, and increased anticipated pleasure for future sessions. Additionally, the gym attendance of these participants was significantly higher, with a 77% increase compared to those who followed traditionally prescribed intensities [20].

These results indicate that when training loads are guided by the perception of pleasure, they can be as effective as traditionally prescribed loads, with the additional benefit of promoting a more positive affective response and greater adherence to exercise programs. This reinforces the importance of considering the emotional aspect in training planning to ensure continuity and long-term success.

Another strategy to apply the concepts of self-determination theory in exercise prescription is to offer participants autonomy, allowing them to choose the intensity of their workouts. Additionally, providing social support, such as engaging in group exercise, can also be beneficial. Researchers have reported an average adherence time of 2 years among participants who received exercise training prescriptions in a small group format (five participants) [21].

A study compared the effects of four aerobic training protocols on the psychophysiological responses of physically inactive adults with overweight and obesity, with an average age of 56 years [22].

Four protocols were analyzed:

Protocol 1: Self-selected intensity, performed individually.

Protocol 2: Prescribed intensity, between 64% and 76% of maximum heart rate, performed individually.

Protocol 3: Small group (three participants), with prescribed intensity (64–76% of maximum heart rate).

Protocol 4: Small group with self-selected intensity.

In the self-selected intensity protocols, participants were instructed to choose an aerobic exercise pace they considered appropriate for their health. The evaluated variables included heart rate, lactate, rating of perceived exertion, perception of pleasure during training, perception of enjoyment after training, intention to repeat the exercise session, and total work volume performed.

The results showed no significant differences between the protocols in terms of heart rate, lactate, and perceived exertion. However, psychological responses such as perception of pleasure, enjoyment, and intention to repeat the training session were more favorable in the self-selected intensity protocols. Additionally, the total work volume was similar across all protocols.

These findings indicate that although participants performed equivalent workloads across different protocols, their psychological perceptions varied. The self-selected intensity protocols were associated with greater pleasure perception, higher enjoyment, and an increased intention to repeat the training session.

Another study conducted by our group, based on the assumptions of the hedonic theory, investigated the psychophysiological responses of trained adults under different HIIT training protocols [23].

The participants had an average age of 28 years and a mean body mass index (BMI) of 24. They performed two HIIT training protocols on a cycle ergometer:

Protocol 1: 1/0.5, with high-intensity intervals of 1 minute followed by 30 seconds of rest.

Protocol 2: 1/2, with high-intensity intervals of 30 seconds followed by 1 minute of rest.

The following variables were evaluated: heart rate, systolic blood pressure, rating of perceived exertion, perception of pleasure, and intention to repeat the training session.

The results showed that physiological responses, including heart rate and systolic blood pressure, were similar between the two protocols. However, the perception of pleasure was 16% lower in the 1/0.5 protocol, indicating that shorter rest intervals were perceived as less enjoyable. Consequently, the intention to repeat the session was 21% higher in the 1/2 protocol compared to the 1/0.5 protocol.

These findings suggest that in HIIT training, longer rest intervals are associated with a greater perception of pleasure, which may positively influence the intention to continue training and improve adherence to the exercise program.

An interesting strategy for HIIT training prescription was evaluated in a study that tested the effect of a protocol called affect-guided interval training. In this protocol, participants performed 60-second intervals, alternating between the highest pleasant intensity and the lowest pleasant intensity over 20 minutes. The study aimed to reduce the discomfort commonly associated with traditional high-intensity interval training, seeking to make exercise a more enjoyable and sustainable experience for practitioners [24].

This approach was designed to minimize the negative sensations that often lead to dropout or lack of adherence to high-intensity training, thereby promoting the continuity of the exercise program.

The affect-guided HIIT training protocol was compared to two other methods: traditional HIIT, with prescribed intensities alternating between high and low, and HIIT with self-selected loads. The results indicated that affect-guided training provided a greater perception of pleasure during the exercise session, while physiological responses (such as heart rate and other indicators) were similar across protocols.

A particularly interesting finding of this study was that affect-guided HIIT not only generated greater pleasure during the session but also led to higher remembered pleasure and a more positive future expectation regarding the performance of new exercise sessions. This suggests that this approach may contribute to greater long-term adherence by making the training experience more enjoyable and inviting.

In order to examine exercise intensity and psychophysiological responses in a self-selected load training group, a study was conducted with 12 sedentary men with an average age of 35 years. They were instructed to choose the load on their own to complete three sets of 10 repetitions in strength training. The group chose, on average, a load equivalent to approximately 55% of a repetition maximum. This intensity is recommended to increase the strength of sedentary individuals who do not practice strength training regularly [25].

Collectively, these studies indicate that self-selection of intensity, in both aerobic and strength training, is an effective strategy for starting training programs, especially for people with low physical fitness, overweight, or obesity. In addition, this approach favors a greater perception of pleasure during exercise and a greater intention to repeat sessions, which can contribute to better adherence and long-term maintenance in physical exercise programs.

Based on the Hedonic Theory of behavior, we can prescribe training intensities based on affective valence. It refers to the feeling of pleasure or displeasure during exercise. It can be a valuable tool for prescribing aerobic exercise. By monitoring how the individual feels while exercising, it is possible to adjust the intensity to maximize feelings of pleasure and minimize discomfort. In this way, the prescription can be customized, keeping the intensity within a zone where the practitioner feels good, which can increase long-term exercise adherence and make the practice more sustainable and enjoyable.

For the prescription of aerobic exercise, we can use the schematic model of the *Felling Scale* proposed below. In this model, the score of 2 and the scores above represent a moderate intensity, which is below the first ventilatory threshold. On the other hand, the score of 1 to "-2" corresponds to vigorous intensity, which is at the point of respiratory compensation. Finally, the scores from plus 2 to "-5" indicate a severe intensity, close to VO2 peak. This model allows adjusting the intensity of the exercise according to the practitioner's subjective perception of pleasure, facilitating the individualization of the aerobic prescription as shown in **Figure 4**.

Obesity associated with sarcopenia, known as sarcopenic obesity, represents a serious clinical problem as it combines low muscle mass with excess adipose tissue, intensifying metabolic and functional risks. Individuals with sarcopenic obesity have greater insulin resistance, chronic low-grade inflammation, and an unfavorable lipid profile, increasing the predisposition to cardiovascular diseases and the development of type 2 diabetes. In addition, the reduction in muscle mass compromises functional capacity, favoring decreased mobility and increasing the risk of falls, fractures, and

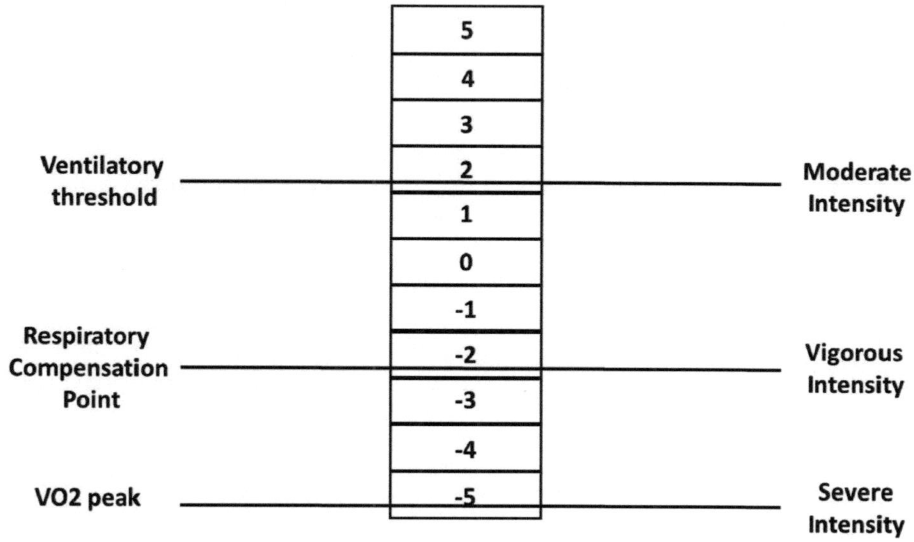

Figure 4.
Schematic model adapted from the Felling Scale *relating the intensities in aerobic exercise [26].*

loss of independence at older ages. The coexistence of sarcopenia and obesity also results in a negative cycle in which limited mobility reduces the practice of physical activities, which further aggravates muscle loss and favors fat accumulation, making it difficult to adhere to weight loss programs [6].

Strength training emerges as a highly effective strategy to reverse the negative effects of sarcopenic obesity, promoting significant gains in muscle mass, strength, and functionality. Unlike aerobic training alone, which can result in additional loss of lean mass when not accompanied by a resisted stimulus, strength training acts directly on the preservation of muscles, stimulating protein synthesis and muscle hypertrophy. In addition, there is evidence that resistance training improves insulin signaling in skeletal muscles, reducing insulin resistance and aiding in glycemic control. Another relevant aspect is its ability to modulate the chronic inflammation associated with obesity through the release of anti-inflammatory myokines that exert beneficial effects on systemic metabolism [6].

To maximize the benefits of strength training in sarcopenic obesity, it is essential to adopt an individualized approach, considering the prescription of exercises that include gradual progression of load, variation of stimuli, and adequacy to the individual's functional capacity. Protocols that involve multi-joint exercises, with moderate to high intensity, performed at least two to three times a week, are indicated to optimize strength and muscle mass gains. In addition, the association of resistance training with appropriate nutritional strategies, such as adequate protein consumption, enhances the anabolic response to exercise and contributes to the maintenance of functionality. Thus, strength training not only combats the negative impacts of sarcopenic obesity but also improves quality of life, autonomy, and longevity, reducing the risk of comorbidities and improving the ability to adhere to sustainable weight loss programs [6].

For the prescription of strength training, one study evaluated the reliability of *the Feeling Scale* for self-selection of intensity in strength training. The results showed that it is a reliable instrument for prescribing strength exercise based on intensity percentages, allowing practitioners to adjust their loads according to the sensations perceived during training. **Table 1** demonstrates the results obtained, highlighting the effectiveness of the scale in determining appropriate intensities for strength training [27].

Autonomy in the choice of training intensities is an essential strategy to improve the experience of individuals who are overweight, obese, and not very physically active, taking into account not only the basic psychological needs of self-determination theory and the principles of hedonic theory, but also the factors of efficacy, safety, and perception of pleasure. Allowing practitioners to choose the intensity of the exercises meets the need for autonomy while promoting a greater sense of control over the training process itself, favoring engagement.

Exercises - % 1 RM				
Feeling scale	**Leg press**	**Leg extension**	**Bench press**	**Elbow curl**
5	43%	37%	42%	39%
3	58%	55%	55%	54%
1	70%	65%	66%	68%
−1	81%	78%	78%	83%

Table 1.
Association of the feeling scale *and % of 1RM for strength training prescription [27].*

The perception of pleasure during exercise is crucial to increasing the intention to continue, as individuals who feel good during the practice are more inclined to repeat the experience. In addition, self-selection of intensity can ensure that exercise is performed within safe and effective levels by practitioners, which is especially important for beginners or people with lower physical fitness.

By combining autonomy with the monitoring of the perception of pleasure, we can create an environment where physical training is perceived as safe, effective, and enjoyable and can contribute to greater adherence and good quality motivation in the long term. Promoting not only physiological results but also a sustainable and pleasurable experience.

A study that explored how motivation can control body weight and impact changes in food choices, exercise, and body mass index (BMI) over time. Their results showed that participants who had a higher perception of autonomy in health-related behaviors, including food choices and physical exercise, lost and maintained the weight lost compared to participants who had a lower perception of autonomy. Autonomous motivation is associated with healthier food choices, greater adherence to physical exercise, and sustained long-term weight loss [28].

4. Conclusion

Adherence to exercise training programs remains one of the biggest challenges faced by overweight and obese individuals. Although the benefits of physical activity are widely recognized, the high dropout rates and the difficulty in maintaining regular practice highlight the need for more effective strategies to ensure exercise continuity. Studies show that it is not enough to prescribe programs based only on physiological and performance criteria; it is essential that the subjective experience of the practitioner be considered as a determining factor in his permanence in practice.

The dual-process theory, the hedonic theory, and the theory of self-determination provide solid foundations for understanding how individuals perceive and react to physical exercise, pointing out that affective valence during practice may be a more relevant factor for adherence than the physical results obtained. Strategies that promote positive sensations during training, such as self-selected intensity, modulation of effort based on the perception of pleasure, and the creation of a motivating environment, are able to generate greater engagement and facilitate the formation of sustainable habits.

In addition, individualization of training is an essential aspect to optimize adherence. Choosing exercise intensity based on the subjective perception of effort and pleasure allows exercisers to adjust their sessions autonomously while respecting their individual preferences and limitations. Evidence indicates that this method does not compromise the physiological effectiveness of the training and, at the same time, significantly improves the practitioner's experience, increasing their willingness to maintain the practice in the long term.

Another determining factor for adherence to physical training is social support. Sessions held in small groups or with the presence of a qualified professional can contribute to a more motivating and welcoming environment, reducing the feeling of discomfort and promoting a sense of belonging. Social interaction and stimulation among participants are important factors in maintaining engagement, especially for individuals who have a negative relationship with exercise.

In addition, strategies such as prescription based on the perception of pleasure and the use of tools such as the Feeling Scale allow you to monitor affective reactions to exercise, providing immediate adjustments in intensity to avoid negative experiences. This reinforces the importance of flexibility in prescribing training, ensuring that it is not only effective and safe but also pleasurable for the practitioner.

The integration of the Hedonic Theory and Self-Determination Theory principles into the training prescription can transform the experience of overweight and obese individuals, making exercise more accessible, enjoyable, and sustainable. Consideration of basic psychological needs—autonomy, competence, and relationship—and adaptation of intensities to the level of perceived pleasure are key approaches to increasing adherence and minimizing high dropout rates.

Thus, a tripartite prescription model, which combines safety, efficacy, and pleasure, may be the key to reversing inactivity rates and improving long-term adherence. The search for the "optimal dose" of exercise should not only focus on maximizing physiological effects but also on creating experiences that individuals want to repeat voluntarily. The new guidelines for the prescription of physical exercise should integrate strategies that consider both the objective aspects of training and the subjective responses of practitioners, promoting a more humanized and effective approach to combating physical inactivity.

Thus, the evolution of exercise prescription practices needs to move toward a model that not only imposes physiological challenges on practitioners but also takes into account their motivation, pleasure, and engagement. By better understanding the factors that influence the continuity of exercise, we can build programs that go beyond the simple recommendation of minutes of physical activity and create a scenario in which exercise becomes part of people's lifestyles, promoting health and quality of life in a sustainable and lasting way.

Acknowledgements

I would like to express my sincere gratitude to the Research Group on Training, Physical Activity, and Health (GETAFIS) and São Judas Tadeu University for their encouragement and support in the development of this chapter. The commitment of GETAFIS to research and knowledge dissemination has been fundamental to advancing science in the field of training and physical activity. The exchange of experiences and the collaborative environment provided by the group were essential for the development of this work.

Furthermore, São Judas Tadeu University has been a key pillar in fostering research and academic production, offering resources, structure, and an environment that values scientific investigation and the application of knowledge in health promotion. Institutional and academic support has been crucial in shaping this chapter, enabling the exploration of new approaches and strategies in exercise prescription.

I extend my gratitude to all professors, researchers, and colleagues who contributed with discussions, insights, and encouragement throughout this process. This work is the result of a collective effort that reflects a commitment to academic excellence and the positive impact of science on society.

Conflict of interest

The authors declare that they have no conflicts of interest related to this work.

Author details

Carlos Eduardo Rosa da Silva*, Diego Santiago, Eduardo Barbosa,
Antonio Roberto Doro, Adriano Verame, Leonardo Lima, Gustavo Almeida,
Wilian Santana and Aylton Figueira Jr
GETAFIS, São Judas Tadeu University, Brazil

*Address all correspondence to: silva_personal@hotmail.com

References

[1] Ekelund U, Ward HA, Norat T, Luan J, May AM, Weiderpass E, et al. Physical activity and all-cause mortality across levels of overall and abdominal adiposity in European men and women: The European prospective investigation into cancer and nutrition study (EPIC). The American Journal of Clinical Nutrition. 2015;**101**(3):613-621

[2] Guthold R, Stevens GA, Riley LM, Bull FC. Worldwide trends in insufficient physical activity from 2001 to 2016: A pooled analysis of 358 population-based surveys with 1.9 million participants. The Lancet Global Health. 2018;**6**(10):e1077-e1e86

[3] Fildes A, Charlton J, Rudisill C, Littlejohns P, Prevost AT, Gulliford MC. Probability of an obese person attaining Normal body weight: Cohort study using electronic health records. American Journal of Public Health. 2015;**105**(9):e54-e59

[4] Cheval B, Boisgontier M. The theory of effort minimization in physical activity. Exercise and Sport Sciences Reviews. 2021;**49**:168-178

[5] Franz M, VanWormer J, Crain AL, Boucher J, Histon T, Caplan W, et al. Weight-loss outcomes: A systematic review and meta-analysis of weight-loss clinical trials with a minimum 1-year follow-up. Journal of the American Dietetic Association. 2007;**107**:1755-1767

[6] Jakicic J, Apovian C, Barr-Anderson D, Courcoulas A, Donnelly J, Ekkekakis P, et al. Physical activity and excess body weight and adiposity for adults. American College of Sports Medicine consensus statement. Translational Journal of the American College of Sports Medicine. 2024;**9**

[7] Garcia-Hermoso A, Lopez-Gil JF, Ramirez-Velez R, Alonso-Martinez AM, Izquierdo M, Ezzatvar Y. Adherence to aerobic and muscle-strengthening activities guidelines: A systematic review and meta-analysis of 3.3 million participants across 32 countries. British Journal of Sports Medicine. 2023;**57**(4):225-229

[8] Sperandei S, Vieira MC, Reis AC. Adherence to physical activity in an unsupervised setting: Explanatory variables for high attrition rates among fitness center members. Journal of Science and Medicine in Sport. 2016;**19**(11):916-920

[9] Dishman R. Compliance/adherence in health-related exercise. Health Psychology. 1982;**1**:237-267

[10] Ekkekakis P, Tiller N. Extraordinary claims in the literature on high-intensity interval training: II. Are the extraordinary claims supported by extraordinary evidence? Kinesiology Review. 2022;**12**:1-14

[11] Ladwig M, Hartman M, Ekkekakis P. Affect-based exercise prescription: An idea whose time has come? ACSM's Health & Fitness Journal. 2017;**21**:10-15

[12] Williams DM, Dunsiger S, Ciccolo JT, Lewis BA, Albrecht AE, Marcus BH. Acute affective response to a moderate-intensity exercise stimulus predicts physical activity participation 6 and 12 months later. Psychology of Sport and Exercise. 2008;**9**(3):231-245

[13] Ekkekakis P, Hall EE, Petruzzello SJ. Variation and homogeneity in affective

responses to physical activity of varying intensities: An alternative perspective on dose-response based on evolutionary considerations. Journal of Sports Sciences. 2005;**23**(5):477-500

[14] Gjestvang C, Abrahamsen F, Stensrud T, Haakstad LAH. Motives and barriers to initiation and sustained exercise adherence in a fitness club setting-a one-year follow-up study. Scandinavian Journal of Medicine & Science in Sports. 2020;**30**(9):1796-1805

[15] Ekkekakis P, Parfitt G, Petruzzello SJ. The pleasure and displeasure people feel when they exercise at different intensities: Decennial update and progress towards a tripartite rationale for exercise intensity prescription. Sports Medicine (Auckland, NZ). 2011;**41**(8):641-671

[16] Marques P, Andrade A, Evmenenko A, Monteiro D, Faria J, Rodrigues F, et al. The preference for and tolerance of exercise intensity: An exploratory analysis of intensity discrepancy in health clubs settings. Current Psychology. 2022;**42**:20629-20637

[17] Deci E, Ryan R. The "what" and "why" of goal pursuits: Human needs and the self-determination of behavior. Psychological Inquiry. 2000;**11**:227-268

[18] Kahneman D, Objective happiness. Well-Being: The Foundations of Hedonic Psychology. New York, NY, US: Russell Sage Foundation; 1999. pp. 3-25

[19] Hardy CJ, Rejeski WJ. Not what, but how one feels: The measurement of affect during exercise. Journal of Sport and Exercise Psychology. 1989;**11**(3):304-317

[20] Teixeira D, Bastos V, Andrade A, Palmeira A, Ekkekakis P. Individualized pleasure-oriented exercise sessions, exercise frequency, and affective outcomes: A pragmatic randomized controlled trial. International Journal of Behavioral Nutrition and Physical Activity. 2024;**21**:85

[21] Wayment HA, McDonald RL. Sharing a personal trainer: Personal and social benefits of individualized, small-group training. The Journal of Strength and Conditioning Research. 2017;**31**(11):3137-3145

[22] Silva CER, Garcia AB, Santana WJ, Pinto LG, Lima LE, Dias HM, et al. Comparison of psychophysiological responses in individual and small group aerobic training with prescribed and self-selected intensity. Preprint. 2023

[23] Verame AS, Santana WJ, Silva CER, Barbosa EJC, Figueira Júnior AJ. Physiological and psychoaffective responses of adults trained in acute hiit protocols. Revista Brasileira de Medicina do Esporte. 2024;**30**

[24] Zenko Z, Hall E, Bixby W. The effects of affect-guided interval training on pleasure, enjoyment, and autonomy: A registered report. Psychology of Sport and Exercise. 2024;**73**:102611

[25] Elsangedy HM, Krinski K, Machado DG, Agricola PM, Okano AH, Gregorio da Silva S. Self-selected intensity, ratings of perceived exertion, and affective responses in sedentary male subjects during resistance training. Journal of Physical Therapy Science. 2016;**28**(6):1795-1800

[26] Bok D, Rakovac M, Foster C. An examination and critique of subjective methods to determine exercise intensity: The talk test, feeling scale, and rating of perceived exertion. Sports Medicine. 2022;**52**

[27] Elsangedy HM, Machado D, Krinski K, Duarte DONPH, Deao GT,

Santos TM, et al. Let the pleasure guide your resistance training intensity. Medicine and Science in Sports and Exercise. 2018;**50**(7):1472-1479

[28] Hartmann C, Dohle S, Siegrist M. A self-determination theory approach to adults' healthy body weight motivation: A longitudinal study focussing on food choices and recreational physical activity. Psychology & Health. 2015;**30**(8):924-948

Chapter 5

Mitochondrial Health in Cardiometabolic Diseases and Aging: Clinical Applications of Therapeutic Fasting and Natural Supplements

Ashutosh Prasad Tripathi, Manish Kumar Verma, Madhulika Tripathi and Brijesh Kumar Singh

Abstract

Mitochondria play a central role in cellular energy production, metabolic regulation, and oxidative stress management. Their dysfunction is a hallmark of cardiometabolic diseases, including obesity, diabetes, metabolic-associated steatotic liver disease (MASLD), and cardiovascular disease (CVD). Mitochondrial decline, characterized by impaired oxidative phosphorylation, excessive reactive oxygen species (ROS) production, and mitochondrial DNA (mtDNA) mutations, also accelerates aging and contributes to cellular senescence and metabolic dysregulation. This chapter explores the essential role of mitochondrial health in cardiometabolic diseases and aging, focusing on emerging therapeutic strategies to restore mitochondrial function. Therapeutic fasting, including intermittent fasting and caloric restriction, has shown significant potential to enhance mitophagy, promote mitochondrial biogenesis, and improve oxidative efficiency. Concurrently, natural supplements such as resveratrol, curcumin, spermidine, and green tea polyphenols including vitamins have demonstrated efficacy in mitigating oxidative stress, preserving mtDNA integrity, and supporting electron transport chain activity. This chapter highlights the therapeutic mechanisms and the potential of therapeutic fasting and natural supplements in addressing mitochondrial dysfunction, offering innovative approaches to manage cardiometabolic diseases, extend healthspan, and combat aging-related disorders. The chapter also discusses the challenges and future directions for translating these findings into clinical practice.

Keywords: mitochondrial dysfunction, cardiometabolic diseases, therapeutic fasting, natural supplements, mitochondrial biogenesis, aging, reactive oxygen species (ROS)

1. Introduction

Mitochondria, often referred to as the "powerhouses of the cell," are essential organelles responsible for ATP production, metabolic regulation, calcium homeostasis, and redox balance [1, 2]. Beyond energy metabolism, they serve as central hubs for cellular signaling pathways, influencing cell survival, apoptosis, and inflammation [2, 3]. This multifaceted nature places mitochondria at the center of cellular and systemic homeostasis, with their dysfunction contributing significantly to the pathogenesis of a wide array of diseases, particularly cardiometabolic disorders and aging-related conditions [4]. Cardiometabolic diseases, including obesity, type 2 diabetes mellitus (T2DM), metabolic-associated steatotic liver disease (MASLD), and cardiovascular disease (CVD), are among the most prevalent global health concerns [4]. Mitochondrial dysfunction in these conditions manifests as impaired oxidative phosphorylation (OXPHOS), excessive reactive oxygen species (ROS) production, and mitochondrial DNA (mtDNA) damage, leading to energy deficits, lipid accumulation, and chronic inflammation in metabolic tissues such as the liver, heart, and skeletal muscle [5]. This contributes to a cycle of metabolic dysregulation and cellular stress, exacerbating disease progression.

Similarly, mitochondrial dysfunction is a hallmark of aging [6]. The mitochondrial free radical theory of aging suggests that ROS accumulation during OXPHOS induces mtDNA damage, resulting in mitochondrial dysfunction and exacerbated oxidative stress [7]. Over time, this self-perpetuating cycle accelerates cellular senescence, tissue degeneration, and age-related diseases [8]. Additionally, aging is marked by a decline in mitochondrial biogenesis and dynamics, further impairing metabolic capacity, immune function, and tissue repair mechanisms [5].

Given mitochondria's pivotal role in health and disease, therapeutic strategies aimed at restoring mitochondrial function have gained significant attention [9, 10]. Among these, therapeutic fasting and natural supplements have emerged as promising, non-pharmacological approaches to mitigating mitochondrial dysfunction. Fasting regimens such as intermittent fasting (IF), time-restricted feeding (TRF), and caloric restriction (CR) enhance mitochondrial quality control by inducing mitophagy and stimulating biogenesis *via* AMPK, SIRT1, and PGC-1α activation. These adaptations improve oxidative capacity, metabolic flexibility, and overall mitochondrial efficiency. Complementing fasting, natural supplements such as polyphenols, flavonoids, and terpenoids target mitochondrial dysfunction through antioxidant activity, mitochondrial biogenesis stimulation, and electron transport chain (ETC) enhancement [9]. Compounds like resveratrol, curcumin, and epigallocatechin gallate (EGCG) not only protect mitochondria from ROS-induced damage but also modulate inflammatory and apoptotic pathways, supporting both metabolic and cardiovascular health [11, 12].

This chapter explores the complex relationship between mitochondrial dysfunction, cardiometabolic diseases, and aging, critically evaluating the therapeutic potential of fasting and natural supplements. By integrating insights from preclinical and clinical studies, it aims to advance mitochondria-targeted interventions as a promising strategy for enhancing healthspan and reducing the burden of chronic disease.

2. Mitochondria: Structure, function, and dysregulation

2.1 Mitochondrial structure and genome

Mitochondria are double-membrane organelles essential for cellular metabolism (**Figure 1**) [1]. The outer mitochondrial membrane (OMM) is permeable to small molecules, allowing exchange with the cytosol, while the inner mitochondrial membrane (IMM) forms cristae that house oxidative phosphorylation (OXPHOS) complexes or electron transport chain (ETC), maximizing ATP production [1, 13]. The intermembrane space plays a key role in proton gradient formation, and the mitochondrial matrix contains enzymes for the tricarboxylic acid (TCA) cycle (i.e., production of reducing equivalents, NADH and $FADH_2$ to sustain OXPHOS), β-oxidation (oxidation of largely saturated fats to produce Acetyl Co-A to feed into TCA), and mitochondrial DNA (mtDNA) [1, 14]. Glucose to pyruvate conversion during glycolysis also feeds into TCA by acetyl Co-A. Reducing equivalents from TCA donate electrons to the electron transport chain (ETC). Proton pumping across the

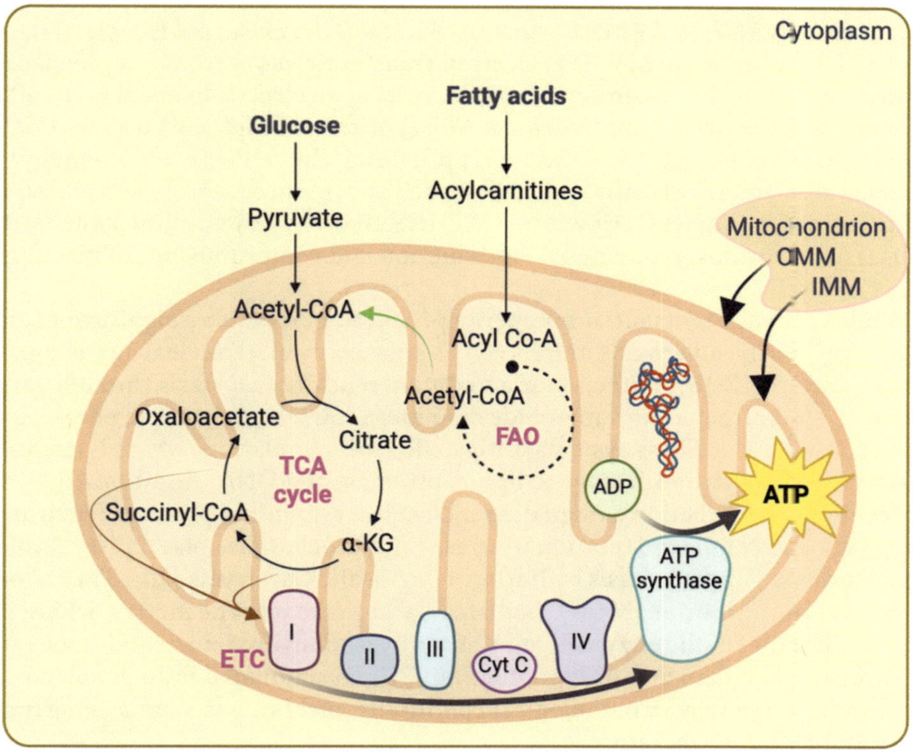

Figure 1.
Mitochondrial structure and core functions: The figure illustrates the basic mitochondrial structure and core metabolic functions within the mitochondrion, that is, fatty acid β-oxidation (FAO), tricarboxylic acid (TCA) cycle, and oxidative phosphorylation (OXPHOS)/electron transport chain (ETC). Acetyl-CoA from glucose and fatty acids fuels the TCA cycle, which donates electrons to the electron transport chain (ETC) to produce ATP. The outer mitochondrial membrane (OMM) facilitates acylcarnitine and other metabolite exchange, supporting bioenergetic homeostasis. Note: the illustration was generated using BioRender.com.

inner mitochondrial membrane (IMM) establishes an electrochemical gradient that drives ATP synthesis *via* ATP synthase, generating cellular energy.

The mitochondrial genome (supercoiled structure in **Figure 1**) is a small, 16.6 kb circular DNA molecule encoding 13 OXPHOS proteins, 22 tRNAs, and 2 rRNAs [1]. Despite its essential role, 99% of mitochondrial proteins are encoded by nuclear DNA and imported [15]. Mitochondria evolved from endosymbiotic bacteria, explaining their independent genome and maternal inheritance. Unlike nuclear DNA, mtDNA lacks histones and has limited repair mechanisms, making it highly susceptible to reactive oxygen species (ROS)-induced damage. Proximity to the electron transport chain (ETC) further increases oxidative stress, leading to mtDNA mutations, impaired energy production, and a vicious cycle of mitochondrial dysfunction [13]. These vulnerabilities contribute to metabolic diseases and aging, emphasizing the role of mitochondria in cellular health [7, 15].

2.2 Functions of mitochondria

The primary function of mitochondria is ATP production through OXPHOS, a process driven by the electron transport chain (ETC) in the IMM [16]. Electrons derived from NADH and $FADH_2$, generated in the TCA cycle, are transferred through ETC complexes I-IV. This electron transfer drives proton pumping from the matrix into the intermembrane space, creating an electrochemical gradient, also known as the proton-motive force. ATP synthase (complex V) utilizes this gradient to phosphorylate ADP into ATP, providing the cell with a high-energy molecule that powers essential processes, such as protein synthesis, ion transport, and cellular signaling [17]. However, OXPHOS efficiency can decline under stress or disease conditions, reducing ATP production and compromising cellular function [17, 18].

While OXPHOS is essential for energy production, it is also a significant source of ROS, primarily superoxide anions ($O_2^{\bullet-}$), formed by electron leakage at complexes I and III [17, 18]. Mitochondria maintain redox homeostasis through antioxidant systems, including superoxide dismutase (SOD), glutathione peroxidase, and catalase [1, 19]. These systems mitigate ROS accumulation, which is critical for preventing oxidative damage to lipids, proteins, and DNA. Additionally, low levels of ROS function as signaling molecules, regulating processes such as mitophagy and cellular adaptation to stress [1]. Mitochondria play a pivotal role in calcium (Ca^{2+}) homeostasis by buffering cytosolic Ca^{2+} levels [20]. The mitochondrial Ca^{2+} uniporter (MCU) mediates Ca^{2+} uptake into the matrix, where it regulates key metabolic enzymes, such as pyruvate dehydrogenase and isocitrate dehydrogenase, enhancing ATP production [21]. Dysregulated mitochondrial Ca^{2+} handling can trigger pathological conditions, including ischemia-reperfusion injury and neurodegeneration.

Mitochondria are central regulators of apoptosis, a programmed cell death pathway critical for tissue homeostasis [22]. During intrinsic apoptosis, pro-apoptotic signals such as Bax and Bak permeabilize the OMM, releasing cytochrome c into the cytosol. Cytochrome c forms a complex with apoptotic protease activating factor-1 (Apaf-1) and caspase-9, initiating the caspase cascade that leads to cell death [23]. Mitochondrial dysfunction, characterized by excessive ROS or mtDNA damage, can dysregulate apoptosis, contributing to pathological conditions such as cancer and neurodegenerative diseases [24].

2.3 Mitochondrial dysfunction in diseases and aging

Mitochondrial dysfunction in metabolic diseases often begins with impaired OXPHOS (**Figure 2**) [25]. ETC inefficiency reduces ATP synthesis, creating an energy deficit that disrupts cellular processes [26]. In insulin-resistant states, such as T2DM, defective OXPHOS in skeletal muscle and adipose tissue impairs glucose and lipid metabolism, exacerbating hyperglycemia and lipid accumulation. In the heart, energy deficits contribute to contractile dysfunction and heart failure [27]. Pathological conditions characterized by mitochondrial dysfunction often involve excessive ROS production [5]. When antioxidant defenses are overwhelmed, ROS react with lipids, proteins, and DNA, leading to oxidative damage [1, 18]. Lipid peroxidation compromises membrane integrity, while protein oxidation impairs enzyme function. Oxidative damage to mtDNA reduces ETC efficiency, perpetuating ROS generation. This vicious cycle contributes to the pathogenesis of MASLD, CVD, and neurodegenerative disorders [11, 26, 27].

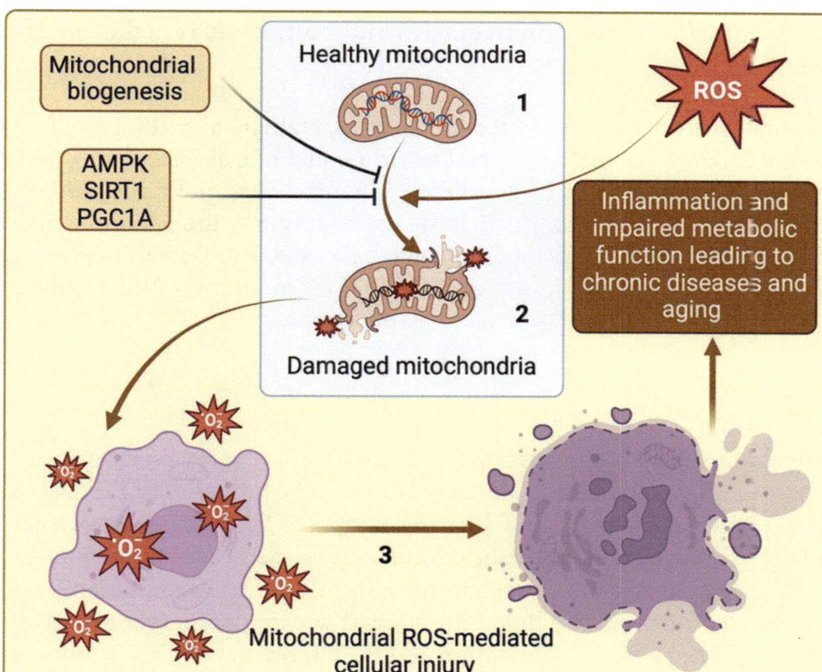

Figure 2.
Mitochondrial dysfunction and ROS-mediated cellular injury in cardiometabolic diseases and aging: The figure illustrates the progression of mitochondrial dysfunction and its impact on cellular health, particularly in the context of cardiometabolic diseases and aging. 1. Healthy mitochondria (indicated with intact inner membrane structures and coupled OXPHOS with normal energy production) maintain efficient ATP production, metabolic balance, and mitochondrial biogenesis, regulated by key pathways such as AMPK, SIRT1, and PGC-1α/PGC1A. 2. Damaged mitochondria exhibit mtDNA mutations, impaired oxidative phosphorylation (OXPHOS), and excessive reactive oxygen species (ROS) production, which drive mitochondrial dysfunction and cellular stress. Strategies activating mitochondrial biogenesis and critical metabolic mediators such as SIRT1, AMPK, and PGC1A inhibit mitochondrial damage. 3. Mitochondrial ROS-mediated cellular injury leads to widespread oxidative damage, promoting inflammation and impaired metabolic functions. These events lead to the development of various cardiometabolic diseases (e.g., obesity, diabetes, and cardiovascular disease) and accelerate aging-related processes, contributing to conditions like neurodegeneration and muscle decline. Note: the illustration was generated using BioRender.com.

Accumulation of mtDNA mutations is a hallmark of aging and metabolic diseases [28]. These mutations disrupt the synthesis of ETC proteins, further impairing OXPHOS [29]. Additionally, age-related declines in mitochondrial quality control mechanisms, such as mitophagy, exacerbate dysfunction [30]. Mitophagy, the selective autophagic removal of damaged mitochondria, is regulated by proteins such as PINK1 and Parkin [31]. Impaired mitophagy results in the accumulation of dysfunctional mitochondria, contributing to cellular stress and metabolic decline [19]. Mitochondrial dynamics, encompassing fission, fusion, and mitophagy, are critical for maintaining mitochondrial integrity [31]. Fission facilitates mitochondrial distribution during cell division and the removal of damaged mitochondria, while fusion promotes complementation between mitochondria, enhancing functional capacity. Dysregulation of these processes leads to fragmentation and the accumulation of defective mitochondria. For instance, excessive fission, mediated by dynamin-related protein 1 (Drp1), has been implicated in MASLD progression, while reduced fusion, regulated by mitofusins (Mfn1/2), contributes to cardiac dysfunction [32, 33].

3. Mitochondrial dysfunction in cardio and metabolic (cardiometabolic) diseases

Mitochondria are central regulators of energy metabolism, making their dysfunction a critical factor in the pathogenesis of cardiometabolic diseases [7, 19, 24, 34]. Altered mitochondrial activity disrupts energy homeostasis, promotes oxidative stress, and triggers inflammatory pathways, contributing to the development and progression of obesity, diabetes mellitus, metabolic-associated steatotic liver disease (MASLD), and cardiovascular diseases (CVD) [35]. This section explores the specific roles of mitochondrial dysfunction in these conditions.

3.1 Obesity

Obesity-induced mitochondrial dysfunction disrupts energy metabolism in adipose tissue and skeletal muscle, leading to metabolic inflexibility [33, 36]. In adipocytes, impaired mitochondrial biogenesis and FAO reduce oxidative capacity, contributing to lipid accumulation. In skeletal muscle, decreased mitochondrial content, ETC activity, and PGC-1α expression impair glucose and lipid utilization [37, 38]. This dysfunction promotes lipid intermediate accumulation (e.g., diacylglycerols and ceramides), triggering inflammation and insulin resistance [26]. Additionally, excess lipids overwhelm mitochondrial oxidative capacity, leading to incomplete fatty acid oxidation, toxic byproduct formation (e.g., acylcarnitines), reactive oxygen species (ROS) production, and systemic metabolic dysfunction [26, 37].

3.2 Diabetes mellitus and insulin resistance

Diabetes mellitus type 2 (T2DM) is characterized by chronic hyperglycemia due to impaired insulin secretion and action, with mitochondrial dysfunction playing a central role [39]. In pancreatic β-cells, defective glucose-stimulated insulin secretion (GSIS) arises from impaired ATP production, reducing the ATP/ADP ratio needed to close K^+-ATP channels and initiate insulin release [38]. In skeletal muscle and adipose tissue, mitochondrial dysfunction disrupts insulin signaling, impairing glucose uptake and driving insulin resistance. Defective OXPHOS increases electron leakage and ROS production, damaging mitochondrial proteins, lipids, and mtDNA [40]. Excess ROS further exacerbates insulin resistance, highlighting mitochondria-targeted antioxidant therapies as potential interventions for diabetes management [18, 26, 41].

3.3 Metabolic dysfunction-associated steatotic liver disease (MASLD)

MASLD, including hepatic steatosis and steatohepatitis (MASH), is driven by mitochondrial dysfunction [42]. Impaired FAO due to reduced CPT1 and acyl-CoA oxidase activity leads to lipid accumulation and energy deficits, sensitizing hepatocytes to lipotoxicity [3, 43]. Dysfunctional mitochondria generate excess ROS, causing oxidative damage, inflammation, and fibrosis. ROS and lipid peroxidation products activate Kupffer and stellate cells, promoting cytokine release and fibrotic remodeling [24]. Additionally, mitochondrial dysfunction impairs mitophagy, leading to the accumulation of damaged mitochondria that further amplify oxidative stress and inflammation [44]. Impaired mitophagy exacerbates mitochondrial damage, while reduced mtDNA copy number and biogenesis drive hepatocyte apoptosis and fibrosis, increasing the risk of cirrhosis and hepatocellular carcinoma [45].

3.4 Cardiovascular diseases (CVD)

Mitochondria are central to myocardial ischemia-reperfusion (IR) injury, where ischemia-induced OXPHOS impairment forces cardiomyocytes to rely on anaerobic glycolysis, leading to energy deficits and mitochondrial destabilization [46]. Reperfusion triggers ROS surges, damaging mitochondrial membranes, ETC complexes, and mtDNA, inducing mitochondrial permeability transition pore (mPTP) opening [47]. mPTP opening causes mitochondrial swelling, cytochrome c release, and activation of apoptotic pathways, leading to cardiomyocyte death [1, 27]. In heart failure, mitochondrial dysfunction reduces ATP production, ETC activity, and FAO efficiency, impairing cardiac contractility [48, 49]. In atherosclerosis, dysfunctional mitochondria in vascular endothelial cells and macrophages generate ROS, activating NF-κB and NLRP3 inflammasomes, promoting inflammation, plaque formation, and cardiovascular risk [50]. These changes accelerate plaque instability, increasing the risk of thrombosis and acute cardiovascular events.

4. Mitochondrial dysfunction and aging

Mitochondria are not only the energy factories of the cell but also central regulators of numerous processes critical for cellular and organismal health [19]. With advancing age, mitochondrial function declines, leading to cumulative cellular dysfunction that underpins the aging process and the development of age-related diseases. This section briefly describes the mechanisms linking mitochondrial dysfunction to aging, with a focus on the mitochondrial free radical theory of aging, age-associated declines in mitochondrial function, and the role of mitochondrial dysfunction in driving age-related diseases.

4.1 The mitochondrial 'free radical theory of aging' and age-related decline in mitochondrial functions

The mitochondrial 'free radical theory of aging' (MFRTA), proposed by Harman in 1972, posits that aging results from ROS-induced damage during OXPHOS (**Figure 2**) [51]. Mitochondria serve as both the primary source and target of ROS, with excessive ROS leading to oxidative damage of mtDNA, proteins, and lipids. ROS, such as superoxide anions ($O_2^{\bullet -}$), hydrogen peroxide (H_2O_2), and hydroxyl radicals ($^{\bullet}OH$), are byproducts of ETC activity [1]. Due to a lack of histones and limited repair capacity, mtDNA is particularly vulnerable to mutations, impairing ETC function and further increasing ROS production [51]. Key studies have demonstrated that mtDNA mutations accumulate with age and correlate with declining mitochondrial function [28, 52]. This self-perpetuating cycle exacerbates mitochondrial dysfunction, bioenergetic deficits, and cellular stress, driving age-related decline. In transgenic mouse models expressing proof-reading-deficient mitochondrial DNA polymerase (Polγ), accelerated accumulation of mtDNA mutations leads to premature aging phenotypes, including hair loss, osteoporosis, and reduced lifespan. These findings highlight the causal role of mtDNA damage in cellular dysfunction, apoptosis, and the aging process [24, 53, 54].

Aging is also associated with dysregulated mitochondrial biogenesis, dynamics, and quality control mechanisms, leading to the accumulation of dysfunctional mitochondria [14, 19]. Mitochondrial biogenesis, regulated by nuclear receptor estrogen-related receptor alpha (ESRRA/ERRα) and PGC-1α, declines with age, reducing mitochondrial density and function [55]. Aging is associated with reduced PGC-1α activity, leading to diminished mitochondrial biogenesis and a decline in mitochondrial density [56, 57]. Mitochondrial dynamics, including fusion (mediated by Mfn1, Mfn2, and OPA1) and fission (regulated by Drp1), are critical for maintaining mitochondrial integrity [4]. However, aging reduces fusion and increases fission, leading to fragmented, inefficient mitochondria prone to ROS production. Additionally, mitophagy, a selective autophagy process crucial for clearing damaged mitochondria, becomes impaired with age [55]. This process is regulated by PINK1 and Parkin, which tag dysfunctional mitochondria for degradation [31]. Age-related declines in mitophagy result in the accumulation of defective mitochondria, further amplifying ROS generation and cellular stress (19Srivastava, 2017 #37). These dysfunctional mitochondria release pro-apoptotic factors like cytochrome c, promoting cellular senescence and tissue degeneration [58].

The accumulation of senescent cells, which exhibit elevated ROS production and a pro-inflammatory phenotype, contributes to chronic inflammation (inflammaging) and tissue dysfunction in aging [59]. This is particularly detrimental in post-mitotic cells such as neurons and cardiomyocytes, which heavily rely on mitochondrial function. Mitochondrial dysfunction impairs ATP production, disrupting tissue repair and regeneration, exacerbating age-related diseases, and promoting systemic decline. Collectively, mitochondrial dysfunction drives the aging process through ROS accumulation, impaired mitochondrial biogenesis, defective dynamics, and insufficient mitophagy, leading to bioenergetic deficits, chronic inflammation, and cellular senescence.

4.2 Mitochondrial dysfunction as a driver of age-related diseases

Mitochondrial dysfunction is a key contributor to age-related diseases, including neurodegeneration, sarcopenia, and cardiometabolic disorders [28, 44].

Neurodegenerative diseases are strongly linked to mitochondrial dysfunction due to the high energy demands of neurons and their dependence on OXPHOS [60]. In Alzheimer's disease (AD), mitochondrial dysfunction is evident in reduced ETC activity, decreased mitochondrial biogenesis, and impaired mitophagy [61]. Amyloid-beta (Aβ) aggregates disrupt mitochondrial membranes, increasing reactive oxygen species (ROS) production, which exacerbates tau hyperphosphorylation and neuronal damage [62]. In Parkinson's disease (PD), mutations in PINK1 and Parkin impair mitophagy, leading to accumulation of dysfunctional mitochondria in dopaminergic neurons, resulting in energy deficits and neurodegeneration [63].

Sarcopenia, the age-related decline in skeletal muscle mass and function, is driven by mitochondrial dysfunction [64]. Aged muscle exhibits reduced mitochondrial content, impaired OXPHOS, and increased ROS, leading to ATP depletion and muscle atrophy [65]. ROS-induced activation of proteolytic pathways, such as the ubiquitin-proteasome system and autophagy, accelerates muscle degradation [66]. Additionally, the decline in mitochondrial quality control results in damaged mitochondria accumulating in muscle fibers, exacerbating metabolic and contractile impairments. Cardiometabolic diseases, including heart failure, atherosclerosis, and metabolic syndrome, are also linked to mitochondrial dysfunction [67, 68]. In the heart, mitochondrial defects reduce ATP production, impair contractility, and promote cardiac remodeling [49, 56, 67]. Aged cardiac tissues exhibit reduced ETC activity, decreased mitochondrial biogenesis, and oxidative damage. In vascular endothelial cells, mitochondrial dysfunction disrupts nitric oxide (NO) production, leading to vascular stiffness and endothelial dysfunction [50]. ROS overproduction activates NF-κB and NLRP3 inflammasomes, driving inflammation and atherosclerosis [69]. In metabolic syndrome, impaired FAO and glucose metabolism lead to lipotoxicity, insulin resistance, and increased risk of T2DM and CVDs [41].

Mitochondrial dysfunction is both a cause and consequence of aging, contributing to cellular senescence, chronic inflammation, and impaired tissue regeneration. The MFRTA links ROS-induced damage to progressive mitochondrial decline. Therapeutic strategies such as caloric restriction, exercise, and pharmacological interventions targeting mitochondrial pathways hold promise in extending healthspan and reducing the burden of age-related diseases. Addressing mitochondrial dysfunction may provide new avenues for promoting healthy aging and improving quality of life.

5. Therapeutic fasting and mitochondrial health

Therapeutic fasting has gathered significant interest as a non-pharmacological intervention to improve metabolic health and mitigate the effects of aging (**Figure 3**). Mitochondria, as the central regulators of cellular metabolism, are profoundly influenced by fasting [70]. By altering energy availability and signaling pathways, fasting promotes mitochondrial adaptation, enhances quality control, and reduces oxidative damage [10]. This section briefly discusses the mechanisms through which fasting impacts mitochondrial health, describes different fasting regimens, and reviews preclinical and clinical evidence supporting their efficacy.

5.1 Mechanisms of action

Fasting enhances mitochondrial quality control, metabolic efficiency, and oxidative stress resistance through several interconnected mechanisms [55, 71]. It promotes

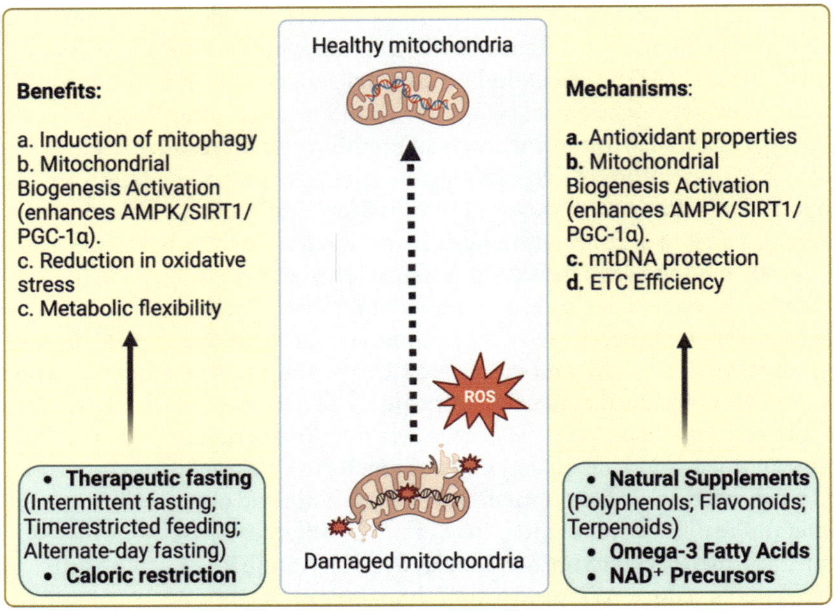

Figure 3.
Restoration of mitochondrial health through therapeutic fasting and natural supplements: The figure illustrates the strategies to reverse mitochondrial dysfunction and enhance metabolic resilience in cardiometabolic diseases and aging. Damaged mitochondria (at the bottom of the central panel) exhibit oxidative stress, mitochondrial DNA (mtDNA) damage, and excessive reactive oxygen species (ROS) production, leading to impaired energy metabolism and disease progression, as shown in **Figure 2**. *Therapeutic fasting (left panel) promotes mitophagy, mitochondrial biogenesis (via AMPK/SIRT1/PGC-1α), oxidative stress reduction, and metabolic flexibility, facilitating mitochondrial renewal. Natural supplements (right panel) such as polyphenols, flavonoids, terpenoids, omega-3 fatty acids, and NAD^+ precursors support antioxidant defense, mtDNA protection, and electron transport chain (ETC) efficiency, improving mitochondrial function. Thus, healthy mitochondria (top of the central panel) represent restored mitochondrial integrity, optimized ATP production, and enhanced metabolic efficiency, achieved through combined fasting and supplementation strategies. Note: the illustration was generated using BioRender.com.*

mitophagy, a selective form of autophagy that removes damaged mitochondria, preserving mitochondrial integrity and preventing oxidative damage. Reduced nutrient availability during fasting activates AMPK and inhibits mTOR, leading to the phosphorylation of ULK1, which initiates autophagosome formation [72]. Additionally, fasting increases the expression of PINK1 and Parkin, key regulators that tag dysfunctional mitochondria for degradation. Studies show that intermittent fasting (IF) enhances mitophagy in skeletal muscle, liver, and heart, reducing lipotoxicity and protecting cardiac myocytes from ischemic injury [73]. Fasting also stimulates key metabolic pathways, including AMPK, SIRT1, and PGC-1α, which regulate mitochondrial biogenesis and energy metabolism [74]. Increased AMP/ATP ratios activate AMPK, enhancing FAO, mitophagy, and mitochondrial biogenesis. Meanwhile, elevated NAD^+ levels activate SIRT1, leading to the deacetylation of PGC-1α, which drives the expression of genes involved in mitochondrial function and ETC assembly. These adaptations improve OXPHOS efficiency, increase mitochondrial density, and enhance cellular energy production.

A key benefit of fasting is its ability to reduce ROS production and oxidative stress, primarily by shifting metabolism toward FAO and ketogenesis, which decreases reliance on glucose oxidation [10]. Fasting also enhances antioxidant defenses by increasing superoxide dismutase (SOD) and glutathione peroxidase activity, which scavenge ROS and protect mitochondrial DNA (mtDNA) from oxidative damage [75]. Furthermore, fasting stabilizes mitochondrial membrane potential, reducing electron leakage and mitochondrial lipid peroxidation, as evidenced by decreased levels of malondialdehyde (MDA) and 4-hydroxynonenal (4-HNE) in caloric restriction (CR) studies [1]. Fasting enhances substrate utilization and metabolic flexibility, allowing mitochondria to efficiently switch between glucose and fatty acids for energy production. It also upregulates ketogenesis, producing ketone bodies such as β-hydroxybutyrate (BHB), which serve as an efficient alternative fuel for mitochondrial OXPHOS, reducing glucose dependency and muscle protein breakdown [76, 77]. Research has shown that fasting increases mitochondrial respiratory capacity in skeletal muscle, improving metabolic flexibility and energy efficiency [78]. Through these mechanisms, fasting optimizes mitochondrial function, enhances metabolic resilience, and protects against age-related and metabolic diseases.

5.2 Types of fasting regimens

Intermittent fasting (IF) involves alternating periods of fasting and feeding, typically on a daily or weekly basis. Common protocols include alternate-day fasting (ADF), 5:2 fasting (5 days of normal eating and 2 days of fasting), and 16:8 time-restricted feeding (16 hours of fasting and an 8-hour eating window) [79]. IF has been shown to enhance mitochondrial biogenesis, reduce oxidative stress, and improve metabolic flexibility [79]. Time-restricted feeding (TRF), a variant of IF, restricts food intake to specific windows of time each day. TRF aligns nutrient intake with circadian rhythms, optimizing mitochondrial function and energy metabolism [79, 80].

Caloric restriction (CR) involves reducing daily caloric intake without malnutrition, typically by 20–40% [81]. CR is one of the most extensively studied interventions for extending lifespan and delaying age-related diseases. CR enhances mitochondrial efficiency, reduces ROS production, and increases antioxidant defenses. Prolonged fasting involves fasting for 24–72 hours or longer, often accompanied by a shift to ketogenesis [82]. Prolonged fasting induces deep autophagy and mitophagy, promoting mitochondrial renewal and metabolic adaptation [71]. Clinical studies suggest that prolonged fasting improves mitochondrial function in individuals with metabolic syndrome and other chronic conditions [81].

5.3 Evidence from preclinical studies

Numerous preclinical studies have demonstrated the benefits of fasting on mitochondrial function in models of metabolic diseases [73, 83, 84]. In obese mice, IF enhances mitochondrial FAO and reduces lipid accumulation in the liver, improving insulin sensitivity [83]. In high-fat diet (HFD)-induced models of diabetes, fasting restores mitochondrial respiratory capacity in skeletal muscle, reducing ROS production and inflammation [83]. CR has been shown to increase mitochondrial biogenesis in the heart and liver, protecting against diet-induced oxidative stress and metabolic dysfunction [73]. In rodents with MASLD, fasting reduces hepatic steatosis by enhancing mitophagy and FAO, while reducing inflammatory markers [83].

Fasting regimens have also been shown to mitigate age-related mitochondrial dysfunction in animal models [79, 85]. CR extends lifespan and preserves mitochondrial integrity in aged mice, partly by maintaining PGC-1α activity and mitochondrial dynamics [86, 87]. Studies in Drosophila indicate that fasting improves mitochondrial proteostasis and delays the onset of age-related neurodegeneration [88]. Prolonged fasting in aged rodents enhances mitophagy and reduces markers of oxidative damage, such as 8-oxo-dG in mtDNA [89]. These findings suggest that fasting preserves mitochondrial function and reduces cellular senescence in aging tissues.

5.4 Evidence from clinical studies

5.4.1 Improvements in insulin sensitivity, lipid profiles, and mitochondrial efficiency in humans

Clinical trials have shown that fasting improves insulin sensitivity and glucose homeostasis by enhancing mitochondrial function [79]. In overweight and obese individuals, IF reduces fasting glucose and insulin levels, increases mitochondrial respiratory capacity in skeletal muscle, and decreases lipid peroxidation markers [80]. CR has similar effects, with reductions in triglycerides and improvements in mitochondrial efficiency observed in humans undergoing a 25% caloric deficit [82]. Fasting-induced ketogenesis also improves metabolic flexibility in humans, enhancing mitochondrial substrate utilization during exercise [85]. In patients with metabolic syndrome, prolonged fasting reduces hepatic lipid accumulation, improves mitochondrial FAO, and lowers inflammatory markers such as C-reactive protein (CRP) [79].

5.4.2 Effects of fasting on cardiovascular health and aging biomarkers

Fasting improves cardiovascular health by reducing oxidative stress, inflammation, and endothelial dysfunction [81]. Clinical studies show that IF lowers blood pressure, improves lipid profiles, and enhances mitochondrial function in endothelial cells [73]. These effects reduce the risk of atherosclerosis and other cardiovascular complications. Fasting has also been shown to influence aging biomarkers in humans [85]. In a study of older adults, CR reduced levels of circulating ROS and improved mitochondrial biogenesis markers such as PGC-1α [90]. Additionally, fasting regimens have been associated with increased levels of circulating β-hydroxybutyrate, a ketone body with protective effects on mitochondrial function and aging [91].

Thus, therapeutic fasting exerts profound effects on mitochondrial health through mechanisms that enhance quality control, reduce oxidative stress, and improve metabolic flexibility. Fasting regimens such as IF, TRF, and CR have demonstrated benefits in preclinical and clinical studies, improving mitochondrial function and reducing the burden of metabolic and aging-related diseases. These findings underscore the potential of fasting as a non-invasive intervention to restore mitochondrial health and promote longevity. Future research should focus on optimizing fasting protocols and elucidating molecular mechanisms to maximize clinical efficacy.

6. Natural supplements and mitochondrial function

Natural supplements derived from plants, marine sources, and other natural origins have emerged as potential therapeutic agents for restoring mitochondrial function and mitigating oxidative stress (**Figure 3**) [5]. These compounds exert their effects through multiple mechanisms, including antioxidant activity, activation of mitochondrial biogenesis, protection of mitochondrial DNA (mtDNA), and improved electron transport chain (ETC) efficiency [92]. This section briefly provides an analysis of the mechanisms of action, key natural products, and evidence from preclinical and clinical studies highlighting their role in enhancing mitochondrial health.

6.1 Mechanisms of action

Natural supplements enhance mitochondrial function primarily through antioxidant activity, mitochondrial biogenesis, and mtDNA protection [92]. Mitochondria generate reactive oxygen species (ROS) as byproducts of electron transport chain (ETC) activity, leading to oxidative damage. Polyphenols and flavonoids, such as resveratrol and EGCG, scavenge ROS and upregulate endogenous antioxidants like SOD, catalase, and glutathione peroxidase. These compounds also activate mitochondrial biogenesis by targeting AMPK, SIRT1, and PGC-1α, increasing mitochondrial density and respiratory efficiency [93, 94]. Coenzyme Q10 (CoQ10) and nicotinamide riboside (NAD^+ precursor) stabilize ETC complexes, reduce electron leakage, and enhance ATP production, supporting mitochondrial health [95].

6.2 Key natural products

6.2.1 Polyphenols: Resveratrol, curcumin, quercetin

6.2.1.1 Resveratrol

Found in grapes and red wine, resveratrol enhances mitochondrial function by activating SIRT1 and PGC-1α. It increases mitochondrial biogenesis, improves FAO, and reduces oxidative damage [96].

6.2.1.2 Curcumin

A bioactive compound in turmeric, curcumin exerts potent antioxidant effects by scavenging ROS and upregulating antioxidant enzymes. It also inhibits mitochondrial permeability transition pore (mPTP) opening, protecting mitochondrial membranes [97].

6.2.1.3 Quercetin

A flavonoid found in apples and onions, quercetin enhances ETC activity, reduces oxidative stress, and promotes mitochondrial biogenesis through AMPK activation [97].

6.2.2 Flavonoids: Epigallocatechin Gallate (EGCG), Catechins

6.2.2.1 EGCG

A major polyphenol in green tea, EGCG reduces mitochondrial ROS production and improves ETC efficiency. It also activates PGC-1α, enhancing mitochondrial biogenesis in muscle and liver [98].

6.2.2.2 Catechins

These flavonoids, present in tea, cocoa, and berries, protect mtDNA, reduce lipid peroxidation, and improve mitochondrial respiration [98].

6.2.3 Terpenoids: Coenzyme Q10, ginseng, Ashwagandha

6.2.3.1 Coenzyme Q10 (CoQ10)

A lipid-soluble antioxidant and ETC component, CoQ10 enhances mitochondrial energy production and reduces ROS generation. It is particularly effective in improving mitochondrial function in neurodegenerative and cardiovascular diseases [99].

6.2.3.2 Ginseng

Ginsenosides in ginseng improve mitochondrial function by increasing ATP production, reducing ROS, and enhancing mitochondrial dynamics [54].

6.2.3.3 Ashwagandha

An adaptogenic herb, ashwagandha increases mitochondrial membrane potential, reduces oxidative stress, and promotes mitochondrial quality control in stress-induced conditions [100].

6.2.4 Others: Omega-3 fatty acids, NAD^+ precursors

6.2.4.1 Omega-3 fatty acids

Found in fish oil, omega-3 fatty acids improve mitochondrial function by enhancing membrane fluidity, reducing inflammation, and activating biogenesis pathways [101].

6.2.4.2 NAD+ precursors

Nicotinamide riboside (NR) and nicotinamide mononucleotide (NMN) restore NAD^+ levels, boosting mitochondrial metabolism, SIRT1 activity, and energy production [102].

6.3 Evidence from preclinical studies

Natural supplements have been extensively studied in animal and cellular models to elucidate their role in improving mitochondrial function in metabolic diseases and delaying aging-related mitochondrial decline. Below, we briefly explore the effects of natural products on mitochondrial health in the context of metabolic diseases and aging, supported by robust preclinical evidence.

6.3.1 Effects of natural products on mitochondrial health in metabolic disease models

Resveratrol, a polyphenol from grapes and red wine, enhances mitochondrial biogenesis in obesity models by activating the AMPK-SIRT1-PGC-1α axis [38].

This increases FAO, OXPHOS, and mitochondrial density. In the liver, resveratrol reduces lipid accumulation, oxidative stress (MDA levels), and insulin resistance while protecting mitochondria from lipotoxic damage by stabilizing membrane potential and reducing mPTP opening [97]. EGCG improves glucose metabolism in insulin-resistant models by enhancing mitochondrial respiration and reducing ROS. EGCG activates AMPK, promotes mitochondrial biogenesis, and improves mitochondrial coupling efficiency, reducing electron leakage [103]. CoQ10 restores ETC activity, ATP production, and β-cell function while reducing ROS and oxidative stress-induced apoptosis [104]. In skeletal muscle, it enhances FAO and mitochondrial efficiency, improving insulin sensitivity [105]. Omega-3 fatty acids (EPA/DHA) increase FAO, mitochondrial membrane fluidity, and ETC efficiency, reducing triglyceride accumulation, ROS production, and metabolic inflexibility in obesity and diabetes models [38].

6.3.2 Delayed aging and improved mitochondrial quality control in animal studies

Curcumin reduces mtDNA oxidative damage by scavenging ROS and upregulating antioxidant enzymes like SOD and glutathione peroxidase [106]. It enhances mitophagy *via* the PINK1-Parkin pathway, facilitating the removal of damaged mitochondria. In aged muscle, curcumin restores mitochondrial membrane potential, preventing atrophy and fatigue [107]. Quercetin extends lifespan in model organisms by reducing mitochondrial ROS and enhancing antioxidant defenses [97]. In aged mice, it activates AMPK, promotes mitochondrial biogenesis, and preserves respiratory function [108]. Quercetin also protects against neurodegeneration in Parkinson's and Alzheimer's disease models, reducing oxidative stress and cognitive decline [109]. NR and NMN restore NAD^+ levels, activating SIRT1 and PGC-1α, driving mitochondrial biogenesis and mitophagy [110]. These effects improve muscle strength, endurance, and cognitive function, countering aging-related mitochondrial decline. Thus, these compounds enhance mitochondrial function, reduce oxidative stress, and promote healthy aging, offering potential therapeutic benefits for metabolic and neurodegenerative diseases.

6.4 Evidence from clinical studies

Natural supplements have gained attention in clinical research as promising non-pharmacological interventions to improve mitochondrial function in individuals with metabolic disorders and to delay age-related mitochondrial decline [111, 112]. Clinical trials provide robust evidence supporting the efficacy of these supplements in enhancing mitochondrial health, reducing oxidative stress, and improving metabolic and functional outcomes. This section briefly provides details on the clinical impact of natural supplements in patients with metabolic diseases and their role in preventing mitochondrial dysfunction associated with aging.

6.4.1 Impact of natural supplements on mitochondrial function in patients with metabolic disorders

Resveratrol has been shown to enhance mitochondrial biogenesis in patients with obesity and T2DM by activating the AMPK-SIRT1-PGC-1α pathway [38, 96]. A clinical trial found that 150 mg/day of resveratrol for 30 days increased PGC-1α expression in skeletal muscle, improved insulin sensitivity (HOMA-IR), and reduced hepatic lipid accumulation [113]. Additionally, resveratrol lowers inflammatory markers (CRP, IL-6), supporting mitochondrial OXPHOS and metabolic homeostasis. Omega-3 fatty acids (EPA/DHA) improve mitochondrial efficiency by enhancing FAO and reducing ROS production. In a 12-week trial, 3 g/day of omega-3s increased mitochondrial respiratory capacity, lowered triglycerides, and improved lipid profiles [114]. Omega-3s also suppress NF-κB signaling, reducing inflammation and mitochondrial dysfunction in the liver and adipose tissue. CoQ10 restores ETC activity and mitochondrial membrane potential in T2DM patients. A 12-week trial using 200 mg/day showed improved glycemic control (HbA1c), increased mitochondrial complex I/II activity, and reduced oxidative stress (8-oxo-dG, MDA levels) [115]. EGCG enhances mitochondrial respiration and antioxidant defenses. A 12-week study (300 mg/day) in overweight individuals improved mitochondrial oxygen consumption, reduced visceral fat, and improved lipid profiles, highlighting its potential in metabolic health [116].

6.4.2 Role in preventing age-related mitochondrial decline

NAD^+ decline impairs sirtuin activation, promoting cellular senescence [110]. Clinical trials show that 1 g/day of NR for 8 weeks increases NAD^+ levels, activates SIRT1, and enhances mitochondrial respiratory capacity, improving muscle strength and endurance in elderly individuals [117]. CoQ10 protects against mitochondrial dysfunction and oxidative damage in aging. Studies show that 200 mg/day of CoQ10 for 12 weeks reduces lipid peroxidation (MDA levels), increases antioxidant capacity, and improves cardiovascular health, muscle strength, and fatigue in elderly participants with sarcopenia [115]. A 12-week trial (1 g/day of curcumin) reduced CRP and IL-6, preserving mitochondrial membrane potential [118]. Quercetin (500 mg/day for 8 weeks) enhanced mitochondrial biogenesis, reduced oxidative stress, and improved physical performance [119]. These findings highlight the potential of NAD^+ precursors, CoQ10, curcumin, and quercetin in preventing age-related mitochondrial decline, improving antioxidant defenses, reducing inflammation, and enhancing metabolic health.

7. Integration of therapeutic fasting and natural supplements

The integration of therapeutic fasting and natural supplements presents a promising avenue for enhancing mitochondrial health, addressing metabolic dysfunction, and mitigating aging-related declines in cellular energy metabolism (**Figure 3**). While both interventions have individually shown efficacy in improving mitochondrial biogenesis, reducing oxidative stress, and promoting metabolic flexibility, their combined application holds the potential for synergistic effects. This section explores the mechanisms underlying these synergistic benefits, discusses translational potential, and outlines future directions for research and clinical practice.

7.1 Synergistic effects

The combination of therapeutic fasting and natural supplements provides a complementary approach to enhancing mitochondrial function, reducing oxidative stress, and improving energy metabolism. Both interventions activate key molecular pathways such as AMPK, SIRT1, and PGC-1α, driving mitochondrial biogenesis and optimizing OXPHOS (**Figure 3**). Fasting-induced activation of these pathways is further amplified by supplements like resveratrol and NAD^+ precursors, which increase NAD^+ levels, improve

ETC efficiency, and support mitochondrial renewal. Additionally, fasting reduces ROS and inflammation, creating an environment conducive to mitochondrial repair, while CoQ10 and curcumin further neutralize ROS, stabilize mitochondrial membranes, and protect mtDNA from oxidative damage. Fasting also promotes metabolic flexibility, shifting energy metabolism from glucose oxidation to FAO and ketogenesis, reducing ROS production and improving mitochondrial efficiency [120]. Omega-3 fatty acids and EGCG enhance FAO and mitochondrial coupling, while NAD^+ precursors optimize ATP production. This synergistic approach improves energy efficiency and reduces metabolic stress, particularly in tissues with high energy demands such as the heart and brain, ultimately helping restore mitochondrial function and cellular homeostasis.

7.2 Translational potential

Despite the promising synergistic effects, translating the integration of therapeutic fasting and natural supplements into clinical practice requires careful consideration of individualized approaches, as well as the challenges and limitations associated with implementation.

7.2.1 Individualized approaches to integrating fasting and supplements

The efficacy of fasting and natural supplements varies based on factors such as age, sex, metabolic health, and genetic background [121–125]. For example, individuals with insulin resistance may benefit more from fasting regimens that enhance insulin sensitivity, such as time-restricted feeding (TRF), while aging individuals may respond better to NAD^+ precursors and CoQ10, which target age-related mitochondrial decline. Developing personalized protocols that consider these variables is essential for maximizing therapeutic outcomes. This may involve tailoring fasting durations, supplement types, and dosages to individual metabolic profiles, which can be assessed through biomarkers such as NAD^+ levels, mitochondrial respiratory capacity, and oxidative stress markers.

7.2.2 Practical challenges and considerations in clinical implementation

The integration of fasting and natural supplements faces several practical challenges:

7.2.2.1 Compliance

Sustaining fasting regimens or adhering to supplement protocols can be difficult for some individuals, particularly those with demanding lifestyles or preexisting conditions.

7.2.2.2 Safety in vulnerable populations

Certain populations, such as pregnant women, elderly individuals with frailty, or those with advanced metabolic diseases, may face risks associated with fasting or high-dose supplements.

7.2.2.3 Drug-supplement interactions

Some natural supplements, such as resveratrol and EGCG, can interact with medications, potentially altering their efficacy or increasing side effects.

To address these challenges, clinical guidelines must emphasize the importance of medical supervision, gradual implementation of fasting regimens, and monitoring for potential adverse effects. Digital health tools, such as wearable devices and mobile apps, can assist in tracking fasting adherence, supplement intake, and metabolic outcomes.

7.3 Limitations, precautions and practical challenges for the integration of therapeutic fasting and natural supplements

The integration of therapeutic fasting and natural supplements as interventions for improving mitochondrial health is promising. However, the practical implementation and clinical application of these strategies are not without limitations and potential risks. Understanding these limitations is crucial for optimizing their benefits while minimizing adverse effects.

7.3.1 Biological variability and individual response

7.3.1.1 Heterogeneous metabolic responses

Individual responses to fasting regimens and natural supplements vary widely due to genetic, epigenetic, and environmental factors. Variations in metabolic flexibility, mitochondrial efficiency, and baseline health conditions can influence the effectiveness of these interventions. For instance: fasting may improve insulin sensitivity in some individuals but could exacerbate glucose intolerance in others, particularly in those with compromised β-cell function. Natural supplements such as resveratrol or NAD^+ precursors may show marked efficacy in individuals with mitochondrial decline but limited benefits in metabolically healthy populations.

Precautions: To address variability, a personalized approach should be adopted. Baseline assessments of metabolic health, including mitochondrial function markers, should guide the choice and intensity of interventions.

7.3.1.2 Sex and age differences

Sex-specific differences in mitochondrial biology and hormonal regulation can influence the outcomes of fasting and supplementation. For example: women may experience different metabolic adaptations to fasting compared to men, partly due to hormonal fluctuations related to the menstrual cycle or menopause. Aging individuals may benefit more from NAD^+ precursors or CoQ10 but could be at higher risk for nutrient deficiencies during prolonged fasting.

Precautions: Tailoring interventions based on age and sex is essential. For older adults, milder fasting regimens and gradual supplementation may reduce the risk of adverse effects.

7.3.2 Safety concerns with fasting regimens

7.3.2.1 Nutritional deficiencies

Prolonged fasting or severe caloric restriction can result in nutrient deficiencies, particularly in vitamins and minerals essential for mitochondrial function (e.g., B vitamins, magnesium, and iron). These deficiencies can impair mitochondrial biogenesis and energy production, counteracting the intended benefits.

Precautions: Fasting protocols should be carefully planned to ensure adequate nutrient intake during feeding windows. Supplementation with essential micronutrients may be necessary, particularly during extended fasting regimens.

7.3.2.2 Risk of hypoglycemia

Fasting can lead to hypoglycemia, especially in individuals with diabetes or those taking glucose-lowering medications. Severe hypoglycemia can result in dizziness, confusion, and, in extreme cases, loss of consciousness.

Precautions: Fasting regimens should be avoided or modified for individuals on hypoglycemic medications. Monitoring blood glucose levels during fasting is crucial for high-risk individuals.

7.3.2.3 Potential hormonal disruptions

Extended fasting periods may alter hormonal balances, including reductions in thyroid hormones, sex hormones, and leptin. These changes can impair metabolism, energy expenditure, and reproductive health.

Precautions: For individuals with thyroid dysfunction or reproductive health concerns, shorter fasting durations or intermittent fasting (IF) with longer feeding windows may be more appropriate.

7.3.3 Safety concerns with natural supplements

7.3.3.1 Overdose and toxicity

While natural supplements are generally considered safe, excessive dosages can lead to toxicity or adverse effects. For instance, high doses of resveratrol can disrupt liver function and lead to gastrointestinal side effects [126]. Excessive omega-3 fatty acid intake may increase the risk of bleeding due to its anticoagulant properties [127].

Precautions: Supplement dosages should adhere to clinically validated guidelines. Monitoring for signs of toxicity, particularly in long-term use, is essential.

7.3.3.2 Drug-supplement interactions

Certain natural supplements can interact with prescription medications, altering their efficacy or increasing the risk of side effects. For example, resveratrol can inhibit cytochrome P450 enzymes, affecting drug metabolism. EGCG can interfere with the absorption of iron and certain medications, such as statins or anticoagulants.

Precautions: A thorough review of an individual's medication regimen is necessary before initiating supplementation. Consultation with healthcare providers is crucial to avoid potential interactions.

7.3.3.3 Variability in supplement quality

The quality of natural supplements can vary significantly due to differences in manufacturing processes, purity, and bioavailability. Contamination with heavy metals or adulteration with unlisted compounds poses additional risks.

Precautions: Supplements should be sourced from reputable manufacturers that adhere to good manufacturing practices (GMP) and provide third-party testing for purity and potency.

7.3.4 Practical challenges in integration

7.3.4.1 Adherence and compliance

The combined application of fasting and supplementation requires long-term adherence, which can be challenging for many individuals. Strict fasting regimens may be difficult to sustain, and daily supplementation can lead to compliance fatigue.

Precautions: Gradual implementation of fasting regimens and simplified supplement schedules can improve adherence. Behavioral support, such as motivational coaching or digital health tools, may enhance compliance.

7.3.4.2 Accessibility and cost

Natural supplements and specialized fasting protocols may not be accessible or affordable for all individuals, particularly in low-income settings. The cost of high-quality supplements, combined with dietary restrictions, can create financial barriers.

Precautions: Efforts should focus on identifying cost-effective fasting protocols and affordable supplement options. Public health initiatives could explore subsidies or support programs for underserved populations.

7.3.5 Population-specific risks

7.3.5.1 Vulnerable populations

Certain populations are at higher risk of adverse effects from fasting or supplementation: fasting may lead to inadequate nutrient intake pregnant and lactating women, affecting fetal or infant development. Prolonged fasting in elderly individuals with frailty may exacerbate muscle loss or worsen nutritional deficiencies. Fasting in individuals with eating disorders can trigger or worsen disordered eating behaviors.

Precautions: Fasting should be contraindicated in high-risk populations unless supervised by healthcare professionals. Alternatives, such as time-restricted feeding (TRF) or mild caloric restriction, may be safer.

7.3.5.2 Individuals with chronic conditions

People with chronic conditions, such as CVD or advanced diabetes, may require modified interventions. Aggressive fasting or high-dose supplements could destabilize their condition or interact with existing treatments.

Precautions: A multidisciplinary approach involving dietitians, physicians, and specialists is essential to ensure safety and efficacy in individuals with chronic illnesses.

7.3.6 Gaps in long-term safety and efficacy data

7.3.6.1 Lack of long-term clinical trials

While short-term studies have demonstrated the benefits of fasting and supplementation, long-term data on safety and efficacy are limited. The potential for cumulative adverse effects, such as nutrient imbalances or organ dysfunction, remains unclear.

Precautions: Long-term randomized controlled trials are needed to establish the safety and efficacy of integrated interventions across diverse populations.

7.3.6.2 Insufficient understanding of mechanisms

The precise mechanisms through which fasting and natural supplements interact are not fully understood. Potential antagonistic effects, such as nutrient depletion during fasting impairing supplement efficacy, require further investigation.

Precautions: Mechanistic studies using advanced techniques, such as metabolomics and mitochondrial respirometry, are needed to elucidate interactions between fasting and supplements.

Thus, while the integration of therapeutic fasting and natural supplements may offer significant potential for improving mitochondrial health and addressing metabolic dysfunction, it is not without limitations and risks. Individual variability, safety concerns, adherence challenges, and the lack of long-term data highlight the need for cautious implementation and rigorous research. Personalized approaches, guided by baseline assessments and regular monitoring, can help mitigate risks. Additionally, future studies should focus on developing evidence-based guidelines, exploring long-term outcomes, and addressing accessibility challenges. By addressing these limitations, the combined use of fasting and supplements can be optimized to maximize benefits while ensuring safety and inclusivity.

7.4 Future directions

To fully harness the potential of therapeutic fasting and natural supplements, further research is needed to address knowledge gaps and optimize their application. Developing reliable biomarkers is essential for assessing mitochondrial health and tracking intervention efficacy. Current markers, such as mtDNA copy number, mitochondrial membrane potential, and ROS levels, provide insights but lack comprehensive assessment. Future research should focus on integrating mitochondrial biogenesis markers (PGC-1α and NRF1), energy metabolism indicators (lactate-to-pyruvate ratio), and inflammation markers. Advanced techniques like metabolomics and mitochondrial respirometry could improve the precision of mitochondrial health monitoring. Optimizing fasting and supplement protocols is crucial to maximizing benefits. Research should explore the effects of different fasting regimens (e.g., time-restricted feeding and prolonged fasting) and supplement combinations (e.g., resveratrol with NAD^+ precursors and CoQ10 with omega-3 fatty acids) to enhance mitochondrial function. Investigating longitudinal effects on metabolic health and aging outcomes is also necessary. Long-term safety and efficacy studies are critical, as prolonged fasting or chronic supplement use may have unintended consequences. Future clinical trials should assess nutritional risks, population variability, healthspan benefits, and disease prevention effects, establishing optimal dose-response relationships. With continued research, fasting and supplementation could revolutionize strategies to prevent and treat mitochondrial dysfunction, promoting metabolic health and longevity.

8. Conclusion

Mitochondria regulate energy production, metabolic balance, and redox homeostasis, playing a crucial role in cardiometabolic diseases and aging. Dysfunctional mitochondria, characterized by impaired OXPHOS, excessive ROS production, and mtDNA mutations, contribute to obesity, T2DM, MASLD/MASH, and CVD, while also accelerating cellular senescence, neurodegeneration, and sarcopenia. This chapter explored therapeutic fasting and natural supplements as mitochondrial-targeted interventions. Fasting enhances mitophagy, mitochondrial biogenesis, and ROS reduction through AMPK, sirtuins, and PGC-1α, while supplements like resveratrol, omega-3 s, CoQ10, and NAD^+ precursors protect mtDNA, improve ETC function, and enhance metabolic flexibility. Together, these strategies synergistically improve mitochondrial resilience, supported by strong clinical and preclinical evidence. Future research should focus on biomarker development, personalized protocols, and long-term safety, integrating these approaches into preventive and therapeutic strategies for metabolic diseases and aging.

Acknowledgements

The authors are thankful to the Ministry of Health (MOH), and National Medical Research Council (NMRC), Singapore, for financial assistance grant number NMRC/OFYIRG/0002/2016 and MOH-000319 (MOH-OFIRG19may-0002), Khoo Bridge Funding Award (DUKE-NUS-KBRFA/2023/0075), and Duke/Duke-NUS Collaboration Pilot Project award (RECA(Pilot)/2022/0060) to BKS; NMRC/OFYIRG/077/2018 to MT.

Conflict of interest

The authors declare no conflict of interest.

Author details

Ashutosh Prasad Tripathi[1], Manish Kumar Verma[2], Madhulika Tripathi[3]*
and Brijesh Kumar Singh[3]*

1 Cardiology Department, All India Institute of Medical Sciences, Kunraghat, Gorakhpur, Uttar Pradesh, India

2 Department of Botany, Raghuveer Singh Government (P.G.) College, Lalitpur, Uttar Pradesh, India

3 Cardiovascular and Metabolic Disorders Program, Duke-NUS Medical School, Singapore, Singapore

*Address all correspondence to: madhulika.triptahi@duke-nus.edu.sg and singhbrijeshk@duke-nus.edu.sg

References

[1] Kakkar P, Singh BK. Mitochondria: A hub of redox activities and cellular distress control. Molecular and Cellular Biochemistry. 2007;**305**(1-2):235-253

[2] Li SY, Gong XY, Ndikuryayo F, Yang WC. The emerging role of mitochondria oxygen redox in pathological progression of neurodegenerative disorders. Ageing Research Reviews. 2025;**104**:102660

[3] Borgne-Sanchez A, Fromenty B. Mitochondrial dysfunction in drug-induced hepatic steatosis: Recent findings and current concept. Clinics and Research in Hepatology and Gastroenterology. 2025;**49**(3):102529

[4] Viloria MAD, Li Q, Lu W, Nhu NT, Liu Y, Cui ZY, et al. Effect of exercise training on cardiac mitochondrial respiration, biogenesis, dynamics, and mitophagy in ischemic heart disease. Frontiers in Cardiovascular Medicine. 2022;**9**:949744

[5] Zong Y, Li H, Liao P, Chen L, Pan Y, Zheng Y, et al. Mitochondrial dysfunction: Mechanisms and advances in therapy. Signal Transduction and Targeted Therapy. 2024;**9**(1):124

[6] Liu X, Zhang X, Zhao L, Long J, Feng Z, Su J, et al. Mitochondria as a sensor, a central hub and a biological clock in psychological stress-accelerated aging. Ageing Research Reviews. 2024;**93**:102145

[7] Balaban RS, Nemoto S, Finkel T. Mitochondria, oxidants, and aging. Cell. 2005;**120**(4):483-495

[8] Spinelli JB, Haigis MC. The multifaceted contributions of mitochondria to cellular metabolism. Nature Cell Biology. 2018;**20**(7):745-754

[9] Liang Z, Currais A, Soriano-Castell D, Schubert D, Maher P. Natural products targeting mitochondria: Emerging therapeutics for age-associated neurological disorders. Pharmacology & Therapeutics. 2021;**221**:107749

[10] Mattson MP, Longo VD, Harvie M. Impact of intermittent fasting on health and disease processes. Ageing Research Reviews. 2017;**39**:46-58

[11] Dhiman A, Handa M, Ruwali M, Singh DP, Kesharwani P, Shukla R. Recent trends of natural based therapeutics for mitochondria targeting in Alzheimer's disease. Mitochondrion. 2022;**64**:112-124

[12] Martucciello S, Masullo M, Cerulli A, Piacente S. Natural products targeting ER stress, and the functional link to mitochondria. International Journal of Molecular Sciences. 2020;**21**(6):1905

[13] Wallace DC. Mitochondrial diseases in man and mouse. Science. 1999;**283**(5407):1482-1488

[14] Nunnari J, Suomalainen A. Mitochondria: In sickness and in health. Cell. 2012;**148**(6):1145-1159

[15] Anderson S, Bankier AT, Barrell BG, de Bruijn MH, Coulson AR, Drouin J, et al. Sequence and organization of the human mitochondrial genome. Nature. 1981;**290**(5806):457-465

[16] Mitchell P. Coupling of phosphorylation to electron and hydrogen transfer by a chemi-osmotic type of mechanism. Nature. 1961;**191**:144-148

[17] Brand MD, Nicholls DG. Assessing mitochondrial dysfunction in cells. The Biochemical Journal. 2011;**435**(2):297-312

[18] Murphy MP. How mitochondria produce reactive oxygen species. The Biochemical Journal. 2009;**417**(1):1-13

[19] Harrington JS, Ryter SW, Plataki M, Price DR, Choi AMK. Mitochondria in health, disease, and aging. Physiological Reviews. 2023;**103**(4):2349-2422

[20] Rizzuto R, De Stefani D, Raffaello A, Mammucari C. Mitochondria as sensors and regulators of calcium signalling. Nature Reviews. Molecular Cell Biology. 2012;**13**(9):566-578

[21] Baughman JM, Perocchi F, Girgis HS, Plovanich M, Belcher-Timme CA, Sancak Y, et al. Integrative genomics identifies MCU as an essential component of the mitochondrial calcium uniporter. Nature. 2011;**476**(7360):341-345

[22] Wang C, Youle RJ. The role of mitochondria in apoptosis*. Annual Review of Genetics. 2009;**43**:95-118

[23] Bock FJ, Tait SWG. Mitochondria as multifaceted regulators of cell death. Nature Reviews. Molecular Cell Biology. 2020;**21**(2):85-100

[24] Vringer E, Tait SWG. Mitochondria and cell death-associated inflammation. Cell Death and Differentiation. 2023;**30**(2):304-312

[25] Fernandez-Vizarra E, Zeviani M. Mitochondrial disorders of the OXPHOS system. FEBS Letters. 2021;**595**(8):1062-1106

[26] Bhatti JS, Bhatti GK, Reddy PH. Mitochondrial dysfunction and oxidative stress in metabolic disorders - a step towards mitochondria based therapeutic strategies. Biochimica et Biophysica Acta - Molecular Basis of Disease. 2017;**1863**(5):1066-1077

[27] Zhou T, Prather ER, Garrison DE, Zuo L. Interplay between ROS and antioxidants during ischemia-reperfusion injuries in cardiac and skeletal muscle. International Journal of Molecular Sciences. 2018;**19**(2):417

[28] Srivastava S. The mitochondrial basis of aging and age-related disorders. Genes (Basel). 2017;**8**(12):398

[29] Sun N, Youle RJ, Finkel T. The mitochondrial basis of aging. Molecular Cell. 2016;**61**(5):654-666

[30] Ashrafi G, Schwarz TL. The pathways of mitophagy for quality control and clearance of mitochondria. Cell Death and Differentiation. 2013;**20**(1):31-42

[31] Pickles S, Vigie P, Youle RJ. Mitophagy and quality control mechanisms in mitochondrial maintenance. Current Biology. 2018;**28**(4):R170-RR85

[32] Chan DC. Mitochondrial dynamics and its involvement in disease. Annual Review of Pathology. 2020;**15**:235-259

[33] Liesa M, Shirihai OS. Mitochondrial dynamics in the regulation of nutrient utilization and energy expenditure. Cell Metabolism. 2013;**17**(4):491-506

[34] Dorn GW 2nd. Mitochondrial dynamics in heart disease. Biochimica et Biophysica Acta. 2013;**1833**(1):233-241

[35] Ahola S. Editorial: Mitochondrial bioenergetics and metabolism: Implication for human health and disease. Frontiers in Molecular Biosciences. 2024;**11**:1468758

[36] Heinonen S, Jokinen R, Rissanen A, Pietilainen KH. White adipose tissue mitochondrial metabolism in health and in obesity. Obesity Reviews. 2020;**21**(2):e12958

[37] Holloway GP, Bonen A, Spriet LL. Regulation of skeletal muscle mitochondrial fatty acid metabolism in lean and obese individuals. The American Journal of Clinical Nutrition. 2009;**89**(1):455S-462S

[38] Jun L, Tao YX, Geetha T, Babu JR. Mitochondrial adaptation in skeletal muscle: Impact of obesity, caloric restriction, and dietary compounds. Current Nutrition Reports. 2024;**13**(3):500-515

[39] Rivera Nieves AM, Wauford BM, Fu A. Mitochondrial bioenergetics, metabolism, and beyond in pancreatic beta-cells and diabetes. Frontiers in Molecular Biosciences. 2024;**11**:1354199

[40] Ayer A, Fazakerley DJ, James DE, Stocker R. The role of mitochondrial reactive oxygen species in insulin resistance. Free Radical Biology & Medicine. 2022;**179**:339-362

[41] Prasun P. Mitochondrial dysfunction in metabolic syndrome. Biochimica et Biophysica Acta - Molecular Basis of Disease. 2020;**1866**(10):165838

[42] Mansouri A, Gattolliat CH, Asselah T. Mitochondrial dysfunction and Signaling in chronic liver diseases. Gastroenterology. 2018;**155**(3):629-647

[43] Sinha RA, Singh BK, Yen PM. Direct effects of thyroid hormones on hepatic lipid metabolism. Nature Reviews. Endocrinology. 2018;**14**(5):259-269

[44] Picca A, Faitg J, Auwerx J, Ferrucci L, D'Amico D. Mitophagy in human health, ageing and disease. Nature Metabolism. 2023;**5**(12):2047-2061

[45] Radosavljevic T, Brankovic M, Samardzic J, Djuretic J, Vukicevic D, Vucevic D, et al. Altered mitochondrial function in MASLD: Key features and promising therapeutic approaches. Antioxidants (Basel). 2024;**13**(8):906

[46] Shao Z, Dou S, Zhu J, Wang H, Xu D, Wang C, et al. The role of Mitophagy in ischemic stroke. Frontiers in Neurology. 2020;**11**:608610

[47] Kalogeris T, Bao Y, Korthuis RJ. Mitochondrial reactive oxygen species: A double edged sword in ischemia/reperfusion vs preconditioning. Redox Biology. 2014;**2**:702-714

[48] Rosca MG, Hoppel CL. Mitochondrial dysfunction in heart failure. Heart Failure Reviews. 2013;**18**(5):607-622

[49] Zhou B, Tian R. Mitochondrial dysfunction in pathophysiology of heart failure. The Journal of Clinical Investigation. 2018;**128**(9):3716-3726

[50] Qu K, Yan F, Qin X, Zhang K, He W, Dong M, et al. Mitochondrial dysfunction in vascular endothelial cells and its role in atherosclerosis. Frontiers in Physiology. 2022;**13**:1084604

[51] Sanz A, Stefanatos RK. The mitochondrial free radical theory of aging: A critical view. Current Aging Science. 2008;**1**(1):10-21

[52] Bratic A, Larsson NG. The role of mitochondria in aging. The Journal of Clinical Investigation. 2013;**123**(3):951-957

[53] Trifunovic A, Wredenberg A, Falkenberg M, Spelbrink JN, Rovio AT, Bruder CE, et al. Premature

ageing in mice expressing defective mitochondrial DNA polymerase. Nature. 2004;**429**(6990):417-423

[54] Zhang Z, Huang Q, Zhao D, Lian F, Li X, Qi W. The impact of oxidative stress-induced mitochondrial dysfunction on diabetic microvascular complications. Frontiers in Endocrinology. 2023;**14**:1112363

[55] Singh BK, Sinha RA, Tripathi M, Mendoza A, Ohba K, Sy JAC, et al. Thyroid hormone receptor and ERRalpha coordinately regulate mitochondrial fission, mitophagy, biogenesis, and function. Science Signaling. 2018;**11**(536):eaam5855

[56] Derbre F, Gomez-Cabrera MC, Nascimento AL, Sanchis-Gomar F, Martinez-Bello VE, Tresguerres JA, et al. Age associated low mitochondrial biogenesis may be explained by lack of response of PGC-1alpha to exercise training. Age (Dordrecht, Netherlands). 2012;**34**(3):669-679

[57] Wenz T. Mitochondria and PGC-1alpha in aging and age-associated diseases. Journal of Aging Research. 2011;**2011**:810619

[58] Tenchov R, Sasso JM, Wang X, Zhou QA. Aging hallmarks and progression and age-related diseases: A landscape view of research advancement. ACS Chemical Neuroscience. 2024;**15**(1):1-30

[59] Martini H, Passos JF. Cellular senescence: All roads lead to mitochondria. The FEBS Journal. 2023;**290**(5):1186-1202

[60] Klemmensen MM, Borrowman SH, Pearce C, Pyles B, Chandra B. Mitochondrial dysfunction in neurodegenerative disorders. Neurotherapeutics. 2024;**21**(1):e00292

[61] Bhatia S, Rawal R, Sharma P, Singh T, Singh M, Singh V. Mitochondrial dysfunction in Alzheimer's disease: Opportunities for drug development. Current Neuropharmacology. 2022;**20**(4):675-692

[62] Zhang Y, Chen H, Li R, Sterling K, Song W. Amyloid beta-based therapy for Alzheimer's disease: Challenges, successes and future. Signal Transduction and Targeted Therapy. 2023;**8**(1):248

[63] Clark EH, Vazquez de la Torre A, Hoshikawa T, Briston T. Targeting mitophagy in Parkinson's disease. The Journal of Biological Chemistry. 2021;**296**:100209

[64] Wilkinson DJ, Piasecki M, Atherton PJ. The age-related loss of skeletal muscle mass and function: Measurement and physiology of muscle fibre atrophy and muscle fibre loss in humans. Ageing Research Reviews. 2018;**47**:123-132

[65] Marzetti E, Calvani R, Cesari M, Buford TW, Lorenzi M, Behnke BJ, et al. Mitochondrial dysfunction and sarcopenia of aging: From signaling pathways to clinical trials. The International Journal of Biochemistry & Cell Biology. 2013;**45**(10):2288-2301

[66] Powers SK, Schrager M. Redox signaling regulates skeletal muscle remodeling in response to exercise and prolonged inactivity. Redox Biology. 2022;**54**:102374

[67] Costantino S, Paneni F, Cosentino F. Ageing, metabolism and cardiovascular disease. The Journal of Physiology. 2016;**594**(8):2061-2073

[68] Sarkar S, Prasanna VS, Das P, Suzuki H, Fujihara K, Kodama S, et al. The onset and the development of

cardiometabolic aging: An insight into the underlying mechanisms. Frontiers in Pharmacology. 2024;**15**:1447890

[69] Peng W, Cai G, Xia Y, Chen J, Wu P, Wang Z, et al. Mitochondrial dysfunction in atherosclerosis. DNA and Cell Biology. 2019;**38**(7):597-606

[70] Tripathi M, Gauthier K, Sandireddy R, Zhou J, Gupta P, Sakthivel S, et al. Estrogen receptor-related receptor (Esrra) induces ribosomal protein Rplp1-mediated adaptive hepatic translation during prolonged starvation. bioRxiv. 2024:2024.01.09.574937

[71] Mehrabani S, Bagherniya M, Askari G, Read MI, Sahebkar A. The effect of fasting or calorie restriction on mitophagy induction: A literature review. Journal of Cachexia, Sarcopenia and Muscle. 2020;**11**(6):1447-1458

[72] Cozzo AJ, Coleman MF, Pearce JB, Pfeil AJ, Etigunta SK, Hursting SD. Dietary energy modulation and autophagy: Exploiting metabolic vulnerabilities to starve cancer. Frontiers in Cell and Development Biology. 2020;**8**:590192

[73] Diab R, Dimachkie L, Zein O, Dakroub A, Eid AH. Intermittent fasting regulates metabolic homeostasis and improves cardiovascular health. Cell Biochemistry and Biophysics. 2024;**82**(3):1583-1597

[74] Price NL, Gomes AP, Ling AJ, Duarte FV, Martin-Montalvo A, North BJ, et al. SIRT1 is required for AMPK activation and the beneficial effects of resveratrol on mitochondrial function. Cell Metabolism. 2012;**15**(5):675-690

[75] Mladenovic Djordjevic A, Loncarevic-Vasiljkovic N, Gonos ES. Dietary restriction and oxidative stress: Friends or enemies? Antioxidants & Redox Signaling. 2021;**34**(5):421-438

[76] Palmer BF, Clegg DJ. Metabolic flexibility and its impact on health outcomes. Mayo Clinic Proceedings. 2022;**97**(4):761-776

[77] Tripathi M, Gauthier K, Sandireddy R, Zhou J, Guptta P, Sakthivel S, et al. Esrra regulates Rplp1-mediated translation of lysosome proteins suppressed in metabolic dysfunction-associated steatohepatitis and reversed by alternate day fasting. Molecular Metabolism. 2024;**87**:101997

[78] Zhang N, Li Z, Mu W, Li L, Liang Y, Lu M, et al. Calorie restriction-induced SIRT6 activation delays aging by suppressing NF-kappaB signaling. Cell Cycle. 2016;**15**(7):1009-1018

[79] de Cabo R, Mattson MP. Effects of intermittent fasting on health, aging, and disease. The New England Journal of Medicine. 2019;**381**(26):2541-2551

[80] Guo L, Xi Y, Jin W, Yuan H, Qin G, Chen S, et al. A 5:2 intermittent fasting meal replacement diet and Glycemic control for adults with diabetes: The EARLY randomized clinical trial. JAMA Network Open. 2024;**7**(6):e2416786

[81] Flanagan EW, Most J, Mey JT, Redman LM. Calorie restriction and aging in humans. Annual Review of Nutrition. 2020;**40**:105-133

[82] Grundler F, Mesnage R, Ruppert PMM, Kouretas D, Wilhelmi de Toledo F. Long-term fasting-induced ketosis in 1610 subjects: Metabolic regulation and safety. Nutrients. 2024;**16**(12):1849

[83] Chaudhary R, Liu B, Bensalem J, Sargeant TJ, Page AJ, Wittert GA, et al.

Intermittent fasting activates markers of autophagy in mouse liver, but not muscle from mouse or humans. Nutrition. 2022;**101**:111662

[84] Li Y, Liang J, Tian X, Chen Q, Zhu L, Wang H, et al. Intermittent fasting promotes adipocyte mitochondrial fusion through Sirt3-mediated deacetylation of Mdh2. The British Journal of Nutrition. 2023;**130**(9):1473-1486

[85] Longo VD, Panda S. Fasting, circadian rhythms, and time-restricted feeding in healthy lifespan. Cell Metabolism. 2016;**23**(6):1048-1059

[86] Lanza IR, Zabielski P, Klaus KA, Morse DM, Heppelmann CJ, Bergen HR 3rd, et al. Chronic caloric restriction preserves mitochondrial function in senescence without increasing mitochondrial biogenesis. Cell Metabolism. 2012;**16**(6):777-788

[87] Martin-Montalvo A, de Cabo R. Mitochondrial metabolic reprogramming induced by calorie restriction. Antioxidants & Redox Signaling. 2013;**19**(3):310-320

[88] Zhang S, Ratliff EP, Molina B, El-Mecharrafie N, Mastroianni J, Kotzebue RW, et al. Aging and intermittent fasting impact on transcriptional regulation and physiological responses of adult drosophila neuronal and muscle tissues. International Journal of Molecular Sciences. 2018;**19**(4):1140

[89] Giorgi C, Marchi S, Simoes ICM, Ren Z, Morciano G, Perrone M, et al. Mitochondria and reactive oxygen species in aging and age-related diseases. International Review of Cell and Molecular Biology. 2018;**340**:209-344

[90] Kyriazis ID, Vassi E, Alvanou M, Angelakis C, Skaperda Z, Tekos F, et al. The impact of diet upon mitochondrial physiology (review). International Journal of Molecular Medicine. 2022;**50**(5):135

[91] Kokten T, Hansmannel F, Ndiaye NC, Heba AC, Quilliot D, Dreumont N, et al. Calorie restriction as a new treatment of inflammatory diseases. Advances in Nutrition. 2021;**12**(4):1558-1570

[92] Schniertshauer D, Wessel S, Bergemann J. Natural mitochondria targeting substances and their effect on cellular antioxidant system as a potential benefit in mitochondrial medicine for prevention and remediation of mitochondrial dysfunctions. Current Issues in Molecular Biology. 2023;**45**(5):3911-3932

[93] Pyo IS, Yun S, Yoon YE, Choi JW, Lee SJ. Mechanisms of aging and the preventive effects of resveratrol on age-related diseases. Molecules. 2020;**25**(20):4649

[94] Singh AP, Singh R, Verma SS, Rai V, Kaschula CH, Maiti P, et al. Health benefits of resveratrol: Evidence from clinical studies. Medicinal Research Reviews. 2019;**39**(5):1851-1891

[95] Kumar P, Singh A, Kumar A, Kumar R, Pal R, Sachan AK, et al. Effect of curcumin and coenzyme Q10 alone and in combination on learning and memory in an animal model of Alzheimer's disease. Biomedicine. 2023;**11**(5):1422

[96] Bejenaru LE, Biță A, Belu I, Segneanu A-E, Radu A, Dumitru A, et al. Resveratrol: A review on the biological activity and applications. Applied Sciences. 2024;**14**(11):4534

[97] Wicinski M, Erdmann J, Nowacka A, Kuzminski O, Michalak K, Janowski K, et al. Natural phytochemicals as SIRT

activators-focus on potential biochemical mechanisms. Nutrients. 2023;**15**(16):3578

[98] Rudrapal M, Khairnar SJ, Khan J, Dukhyil AB, Ansari MA, Alomary MN, et al. Dietary polyphenols and their role in oxidative stress-induced human diseases: Insights into protective effects, antioxidant potentials and mechanism(s) of action. Frontiers in Pharmacology. 2022;**13**:806470

[99] Noh YH, Kim KY, Shim MS, Choi SH, Choi S, Ellisman MH, et al. Inhibition of oxidative stress by coenzyme Q10 increases mitochondrial mass and improves bioenergetic function in optic nerve head astrocytes. Cell Death & Disease. 2013;**4**(10):e820

[100] Mikulska P, Malinowska M, Ignacyk M, Szustowski P, Nowak J, Pesta K, et al. Ashwagandha (Withania somnifera)-current research on the health-promoting activities: A narrative review. Pharmaceutics. 2023;**15**(4):1057

[101] De Boer AA, Monk JM, Liddle DM, Hutchinson AL, Power KA, Ma DW, et al. Fish-oil-derived n-3 polyunsaturated fatty acids reduce NLRP3 inflammasome activity and obesity-related inflammatory cross-talk between adipocytes and CD11b(+) macrophages. The Journal of Nutritional Biochemistry. 2016;**34**:61-72

[102] Yau WW, Chen GB, Zhou J, Francisco JC, Thimmukonda NK, Li S, et al. Nicotinamide riboside rescues dysregulated glycolysis and fatty acid beta-oxidation in a human hepatic cell model of citrin deficiency. Human Molecular Genetics. 2023;**32**(11):1922-1931

[103] James A, Wang K, Wang Y. Therapeutic activity of green tea Epigallocatechin-3-Gallate on metabolic diseases and non-alcoholic fatty liver diseases: The current updates. Nutrients. 2023;**15**(13):3022

[104] Cirilli I, Damiani E, Dludla PV, Hargreaves I, Marcheggiani F, Millichap LE, et al. Role of coenzyme Q(10) in health and disease: An update on the last 10 years (2010-2020). Antioxidants (Basel). 2021;**10**(8):1325

[105] Xu Z, Huo J, Ding X, Yang M, Li L, Dai J, et al. Coenzyme Q10 improves lipid metabolism and ameliorates obesity by regulating CaMKII-mediated PDE4 inhibition. Scientific Reports. 2017;7(1):8253

[106] Sathyabhama M, Priya Dharshini LC, Karthikeyan A, Kalaiselvi S, Min T. The credible role of curcumin in oxidative stress-mediated mitochondrial dysfunction in mammals. Biomolecules. 2022;**12**(10):1405

[107] Saud Gany SL, Chin KY, Tan JK, Aminuddin A, Makpol S. Curcumin as a therapeutic agent for sarcopenia. Nutrients. 2023;**15**(11):2526

[108] Wang WW, Han R, He HJ, Li J, Chen SY, Gu Y, et al. Administration of quercetin improves mitochondria quality control and protects the neurons in 6-OHDA-lesioned Parkinson's disease models. Aging (Albany NY). 2021;**13**(8):11738-11751

[109] Alsaleem MA, Al-Kuraishy HM, Al-Gareeb AI, Albuhadily AK, Alrouji M, Yassen ASA, et al. Molecular signaling pathways of quercetin in Alzheimer's disease: A promising arena. Cellular and Molecular Neurobiology. 2024;**45**(1):8

[110] Iqbal T, Nakagawa T. The therapeutic perspective of NAD(+) precursors in age-related diseases. Biochemical and Biophysical Research Communications. 2024;**702**:149590

[111] Nicolson GL. Mitochondrial dysfunction and chronic disease: Treatment with natural supplements. Integrative Medicine (Encinitas, Calif.). 2014;**13**(4):35-43

[112] Valero T. Mitochondrial biogenesis: Pharmacological approaches. Current Pharmaceutical Design. 2014;**20**(35):5507-5509

[113] Timmers S, Konings E, Bilet L, Houtkooper RH, van de Weijer T, Goossens GH, et al. Calorie restriction-like effects of 30 days of resveratrol supplementation on energy metabolism and metabolic profile in obese humans. Cell Metabolism. 2011;**14**(5):612-622

[114] Logan SL, Spriet LL. Omega-3 fatty acid supplementation for 12 weeks increases resting and exercise metabolic rate in healthy community-dwelling older females. PLoS One. 2015;**10**(12):e0144828

[115] Akbari Fakhrabadi M, Zeinali Ghotrom A, Mozaffari-Khosravi H, Hadi Nodoushan H, Nadjarzadeh A. Effect of coenzyme Q10 on oxidative stress, glycemic control and inflammation in diabetic neuropathy: A double blind randomized clinical trial. International Journal for Vitamin and Nutrition Research. 2014;**84**(5-6):252-260

[116] Luk HY, Appell C, Chyu MC, Chen CH, Wang CY, Yang RS, et al. Impacts of green tea on joint and skeletal muscle health: Prospects of translational nutrition. Antioxidants (Basel). 2020;**9**(11):1050

[117] Elhassan YS, Kluckova K, Fletcher RS, Schmidt MS, Garten A, Doig CL, et al. Nicotinamide riboside augments the aged human skeletal muscle NAD(+) metabolome and induces transcriptomic and anti-inflammatory signatures. Cell Reports. 2019;**28**(7):1717-28 e6

[118] Alam MS, Anwar MJ, Maity MK, Azam F, Jaremko M, Emwas AH. The dynamic role of curcumin in mitigating human illnesses: Recent advances in therapeutic applications. Pharmaceuticals (Basel). 2024;**17**(12):1674

[119] Kurtz JA, Vandusseldorp TA, Uken B, Otis J. Quercetin in sports and exercise: A review. International Journal of Exercise Science. 2023;**16**(2):1334-1384

[120] Smith RL, Soeters MR, Wust RCI, Houtkooper RH. Metabolic flexibility as an adaptation to energy resources and requirements in health and disease. Endocrine Reviews. 2018;**39**(4):489-517

[121] Cienfuegos S, Corapi S, Gabel K, Ezpeleta M, Kalam F, Lin S, et al. Effect of intermittent fasting on reproductive hormone levels in females and males: A review of human trials. Nutrients. 2022;**14**(11):2343

[122] Soeters MR, Sauerwein HP, Groener JE, Aerts JM, Ackermans MT, Glatz JF, et al. Gender-related differences in the metabolic response to fasting. The Journal of Clinical Endocrinology and Metabolism. 2007;**92**(9):3646-3652

[123] Kouvari M, Panagiotakos DB. Vitamin D status, gender and cardiovascular diseases: A systematic review of prospective epidemiological studies. Expert Review of Cardiovascular Therapy. 2019;**17**(7):545-555

[124] Stjernberg L, Berglund J, Halling A. Age and gender effect on the use of herbal medicine products and food supplements among the elderly. Scandinavian Journal of Primary Health Care. 2006;**24**(1):50-55

[125] Torres P, Cacabelos D, Pairada J, Bauer KC, Boada J, Fontdevila L, et al.

Gender-specific beneficial effects of docosahexaenoic acid dietary supplementation in G93A-SOD1 amyotrophic lateral sclerosis mice. Neurotherapeutics. 2020;**17**(1):269-281

[126] Brown VA, Patel KR, Viskaduraki M, Crowell JA, Perloff M, Booth TD, et al. Repeat dose study of the cancer chemopreventive agent resveratrol in healthy volunteers: Safety, pharmacokinetics, and effect on the insulin-like growth factor axis. Cancer Research. 2010;**70**(22):9003-9011

[127] Gross BW, Gillio M, Rinehart CD, Lynch CA, Rogers FB. Omega-3 fatty acid supplementation and warfarin: A lethal combination in traumatic brain injury. Journal of Trauma Nursing. 2017;**24**(1):15-18

Section 3

Advanced Therapeutic Approaches for Obesity Care

Chapter 6

The One-Anastomosis Gastric Bypass Procedure for Severe Obesity: Technical Aspects and Early Outcomes

Mohamad Hamoud

Abstract

Overweight and obesity have become widespread in Western populations. In the US, obesity rates have been rising for decades, posing significant public health concerns. Data from the CDC and medical journals confirm this steady increase over the past 30 years. Obesity is a chronic, progressive disease affecting multiple body systems, increasing the risk of physical and mental illnesses. Bariatric and metabolic surgeries encompass various procedures designed to treat obesity and its associated conditions. These surgeries, performed for decades in the US and abroad, utilize different mechanisms for weight loss: restrictive surgery, which reduces stomach volume, and malabsorptive surgery, which alters absorption and intestinal hormone effects on satiety, or a combination of both. Bariatric surgery is a complex process with lasting clinical and psychological impacts. Ensuring surgical success requires proper preoperative preparation and postoperative support. Studies indicate that multidisciplinary post-surgical care significantly improves long-term outcomes. Recent evidence suggests that metabolic bariatric surgery may effectively treat type 2 diabetes. The demand for revision surgeries is rising globally, including in the US. Common reasons include inadequate weight loss, weight regain, and correction of complications.

Keywords: one-anastomosis gastric bypass, severe obesity, bariatric surgery, early complication, late complications

1. Introduction

Bariatric surgery has historical roots dating back centuries. Reports suggest early surgical interventions in ancient Rome, Greece, and Spain during the tenth century [1–6]. In the eighteenth and nineteenth centuries, experimental weight-loss surgeries had high mortality rates.

2. Twentieth-century advancements

The first metabolic surgery, the jejuno-ileal bypass, was performed by Kremen in 1954 [7]. Despite limited success due to complications, this era saw the development of more effective procedures like gastric bypass and gastric banding.

3. Late twentieth to early twenty-first century

Advances in laparoscopic techniques made bariatric procedures safer and more accessible, leading to widespread adoption. Today, bariatric surgery is a well-established, effective treatment for obesity and related health conditions.

4. Key milestones

See **Table 1**.

Event	Year
Kremen et al. perform the first jejuno-ileal bypass.	1954
Mason et al. conduct the first gastric bypass surgery.	1967
L. H. Wilkinson performs Nissen's fundoplication with gastric wrapping.	1976
Nicola Scopirano introduces biliopancreatic diversion.	1979
Mason develops vertical banded gastroplasty.	1982
Kuzmak introduces an adjustable gastric band.	1986
Sleeve gastrectomy and other procedures gain popularity [7].	Twenty-first century

Table 1.
Selected significant events and innovations in the history of bariatric surgery.

Bariatric surgery has come a long way since its early days. It is now a safe and effective treatment option for many people with obesity, and it continues to evolve as new techniques and technologies are developed [8].

5. Types of bariatric surgery

Bariatric surgeries reduce stomach size and bypass parts of the intestine, promoting weight loss by restricting food intake and altering nutrient absorption. Over the past decade, metabolic surgery has become more popular. Six types, including the One-Anastomosis Gastric Bypass (OAGB), are now endorsed by global surgical societies. The OAGB, initially developed in 1997, has shown excellent weight loss and improvement in metabolic conditions like diabetes [9, 10].

6. Common types of surgery

Gastric banding: Creates a small stomach pouch, limiting food intake. Adjustable and reversible, but complications like band slippage can occur.

Sleeve gastrectomy: Removes a large portion of the stomach, reducing capacity and hunger hormones. It is the most common procedure today. While effective, it is not without risks like long-term complications [11].

Biliopancreatic Diversion with Duodenal Switch (BPD-DS): For severe obesity, this procedure includes both stomach reduction and bypassing part of the intestine, leading to significant weight loss and resolution of type 2 diabetes. However, it carries risks like malabsorption and nutrient deficiencies [12, 13].

Gallstones: Increased risk of gallstone formation [3].

SADI (Single Anastomosis Duodenal-Ileal Bypass): Combines stomach reduction and intestinal bypass with fewer connections than traditional duodenal switch procedures. It promotes substantial weight loss but also carries risks of malabsorption and nutrient deficiencies [14].

Roux-en-Y Gastric Bypass (RYGB): One of the most effective types, RYGB reduces stomach size and reroutes the intestines, helping with weight loss and improving related conditions. However, it comes with complications like internal hernia and leakage [15].

7. One-anastomosis gastric bypass (OAGB)

Developed by Dr. Rutledge in 1997, OAGB has become a popular choice due to its simplicity and effectiveness. It involves creating a small gastric pouch and bypassing

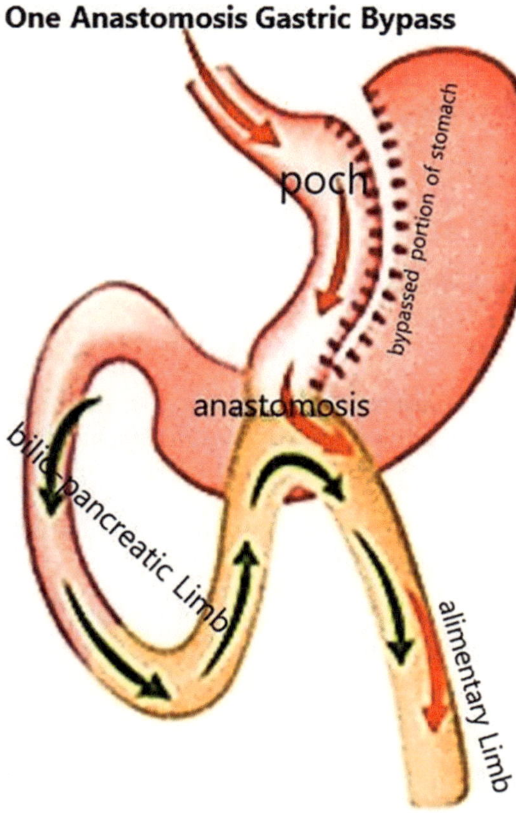

Figure 1.
Diagram of anastomosis gastric bypass.

part of the jejunum, resulting in fat malabsorption. This procedure has gained global support for its rapid, safe, and effective results [16].

One-anastomosis gastric bypass is gaining attention as a standalone bariatric procedure, with surgeons worldwide publishing their experiences. It shows promising results in terms of effective weight loss, comorbidity resolution, and acceptable complication rates in the short and medium term. Proponents argue that it is safer and easier than the gold standard Roux-en-Y gastric bypass (**Figure 1**) [17].

This document outlines the updated guidelines from the Israeli Ministry of Health for performing metabolic and bariatric surgery in adults, specifically focusing on the one-anastomosis gastric bypass.

8. Bariatric surgery center requirements

- *Multidisciplinary team:* The hospital must have a specialized team including:
  - o *Bariatric surgeon*
  - o *Nutritionist*
  - o *Psychologist/social worker*
  - o *Psychiatrist (if needed)*
  - o *Clinical pharmacist*
  - o *Endocrinologist/internist*
  - o *Anesthesiologist*
  - o *Intensive care unit*
  - o Gastroenterology institute
  - o Imaging department
- *Experience:* The center must have performed at least 100 bariatric surgeries annually for the past 5 years, using at least two surgical techniques, and handle repeat/corrective surgeries.
- *Data reporting:* The center must report patient data to the national registry at the National Center for Disease Control.

9. Preoperative preparation process

- Referral and initial assessment:
  - o *Referral from a family doctor after consultation with a bariatric surgeon.*
  - o *Verification that the patient has not refused surgery in the past year.*
  - o *Family doctor assesses Body Mass Index (BMI) and comorbidities.*

- *Required tests and assessments:*
    - *Blood tests (cell count, liver/kidney function, coagulation, glucose, lipids, thyroid, vitamins).*
    - *Gastroscopy/upper GI x-ray, abdominal ultrasound, chest x-ray, ECG.*
    - *Echocardiogram/stress test (if needed).*
    - *Bone density for repeat bariatric surgery.*
    - *Nutritional assessment (at least three sessions over 6 weeks).*
    - *Additional tests as needed (lung function, etc.).*
    - *Geriatric consultation (for patients over 75).*
    - *Anesthesia pre-assessment.*
    - *Psychiatric evaluation (if needed).*
- *Bariatric committee:*
    - *Committee approval is required for surgery.*
    - *Nutritional and psychosocial evaluations are performed.*
    - *Medication assessment.*
    - *Refusal is valid for 1 year.*
- *Appeal process:*
    - *An appeal committee exists for refused cases.*

10. Indications for bariatric surgery

- *BMI ≥ 40 kg/m*^{2}.
- *BMI ≥ 35 kg/m*^{2} *with comorbidities:*
    - *Type 2 diabetes.*
    - *Uncontrolled hypertension.*
    - *Ischemic heart disease.*
    - *Dyslipidemia.*
    - *Sleep apnea.*

- *Reproductive disorders.*
- *Orthopedic problems.*
- *Fatty liver.*
- *Thromboembolic event.*
- *Pseudotumor cerebri.*

- BMI 30–35 kg/m^2:
  - Previous failed bariatric surgery.
  - Uncontrolled type 2 diabetes (HbA1C $\geq$ 8% for 2 years).
- Regardless of BMI:
  - Reoperation after surgical complications.

11. Preoperative nutritional preparation and assessment

- *Detailed assessment of medical history, eating habits, and nutritional status.*
- *Education and counseling on post-surgery dietary and lifestyle changes.*
- *Preoperative weight loss, correction of nutritional deficiencies.*

12. Psychiatric assessment

12.1 Introduction

Bariatric surgery offers significant weight loss, improving health and quality of life. However, success relies on behavioral, nutritional, and emotional adjustments. While many experience positive changes, others may face worsening mental health, including depression and even suicide. Studies show that some patients experience severe depression post-surgery, with higher rates of self-harm and suicidal attempts compared to non-surgical patients [18, 19]. Postoperative pathological eating patterns, whether de novo or a recurrence of previous patterns, are significantly associated with weight regain after surgery [20]. Furthermore, there are cases of patients developing severe eating disorders after surgery, including anorexia nervosa, atypical anorexia, and bulimia nervosa [21, 22].

12.2 Postoperative eating disorders

Candidates for bariatric surgery often show higher rates of eating disorders, particularly binge eating disorder (BED). These patterns, whether new or recurring, are associated with weight regain. Some patients also develop severe conditions like anorexia or bulimia post-surgery [21].

12.3 Psychopathology contraindications for bariatric surgery

1. Untreated or unstable mental state
2. *Conditions in the past year:*
    a. *Active psychosis*
    b. *Suicidal risk or self-harm*
    c. *Severe major depression*
    d. *Substance or alcohol abuse*
    e. *Acute stressors affecting health*
    f. *Cognitive impairment affecting consent or post-surgery compliance*
3. Active eating disorder
4. Patient misunderstanding of risks, benefits, or alternatives

13. Lack of commitment to supplements and long-term follow-up

13.1 Psychosocial assessment

Evaluation of personal history, eating behaviors, readiness for surgery, support systems, and mental health.

13.2 Contraindications for bariatric surgery

Summarizes psychiatric contraindications.
Medical contraindications (malignancy, pregnancy).

13.3 Key takeaways

The guidelines emphasize a multidisciplinary approach and rigorous preoperative evaluations.
Psychiatric and nutritional assessments are crucial for patient selection and success.
Specific BMI and comorbidity criteria are outlined for surgery eligibility.
A clear process for appeal is provided for patients who are refused surgery.

14. Standardization of the one-anastomosis gastric bypass procedure: Study overview

14.1 Study setting

Conducted at the Surgical Department, Holy Family Hospital, Nazareth [20].
Study design:
Retrospective database analysis: Researchers analyzed pre-existing patient data.

Prospectively maintained database: Data was systematically recorded during treatment, ensuring accuracy.
Single bariatric center: Consistent surgical techniques, but findings may not be broadly generalizable.
No IRB approval required: As a retrospective chart review, formal IRB approval was deemed unnecessary.
Inclusion and exclusion criteria.
Inclusion criteria:
Timeframe: Patients who underwent OAGB surgery between January 2016 and December 2021.
Age: Between 18 and 65 years old.
Obesity:
Severe obesity (Class III) with BMI $\geq$ 40.0 kg/m^2 or.
Moderate obesity (Class II) with BMI $\geq$ 35.0 kg/m^2 and at least one comorbidity.
Informed consent: Patients must have provided informed consent before surgery.
Follow-up data: Complete 30-day postoperative follow-up data.
Exclusion criteria:
Mental health: Excluded patients with poorly controlled mental illnesses.
Pregnancy/Lactation: Excluded pregnant or breastfeeding women.

14.2 Postoperative care protocol

- *Drainage: Closed suction drain placed near the staple line to monitor for leaks or bleeding.*

- *Imaging: No routine upper GI imaging post-surgery.*

- *Oral intake and discharge: Resumed on the first day, with discharge typically on day two.*

- *DVT prevention: Low-molecular-weight heparin administered for 10 days post-surgery.*

- *Acid suppression: Proton pump inhibitors (PPIs) prescribed for 6 months.*

- *Follow-up schedule: First appointment 10 days post-surgery, with subsequent visits at 3, 6, 12, and 24 months.*

14.3 Statistical analysis

Software: SPSS version 28.0.
Data presentation:
Continuous variables: Presented as means ± standard deviations.
Categorical variables: Presented as frequencies and percentages.
Normality testing: Kolmogorov-Smirnov test.
Tests used:
Independent samples t-test for normally distributed data.
Mann-Whitney U test for non-normally distributed data.
Chi-squared test for categorical variables.
Statistical significance: p-value <0.05.

14.4 Results

- *Patient population:* 775 patients, with 774 analyzed after excluding one for missing data.
- *Follow-up:* Complete 30-day follow-up data available for all 774 patients.
- *Trend:* Annual OAGB procedures increased from 66 in 2016 to 191 in 2021 (189% increase).
- *Statistical significance:* Increase in procedures was statistically significant ($p < 0.05$) (**Table 2**).

14.5 Patient characteristics

- *Gender: 83.6% female (647 patients).*
- *Age: Average age 36.2 years (SD: 10.8 years), ranging from 18 to 70 years. Only 12.1% (94 patients) were 50 years or older.*
- *BMI: Average BMI of 42.7 kg/m^2 (SD: 4.2 kg/m^2), ranging from 17.2 to 61.0 kg/m^2. Six percent of patients (46 individuals) had a BMI ≥ 50 kg/m^2.*
- *Weight: Average weight of 115.5 kg (SD: 16.5 kg), ranging from 48.0 kg to 182.0 kg* (**Table 3**)

The study primarily consisted of younger women with severe obesity, though a range of BMIs and weights were represented.

1. Statistical comparison:
2. Statistical tests: The Mann-Whitney test, a non-parametric method for comparing groups with non-normally distributed data, and the chi-squared (χ^2) test for categorical data (e.g., complications) were used to determine statistical significance.

Year	No. procedures [n (%)]
2016	66 (8.5)
2017	112 (14.5)
2018	124 (16.0)
2019	133 (17.2)
2020	148 (19.1)
2021	191 (24.7)
Total (2016–2021)	774 (100.0)

Table 2.
Number of one-anastomosis gastric bypass procedures performed per year between 2016 and 2021.

Characteristics	Total OAGB population (N = 774)	Primary OAGB (n = 681)	Revisional OAGB (n = 93)	*P*‡
Age [mean ± SD (range)] (y)	36.2 ± 10.8 (18.0–70)	35.5 ± 10.6	41.8 ± 10.1	<0.001
Age > 50 (y)	94 (12.1)	75 (11.0)	19 (20.4)	0.016
Weight [mean ± SD (range)] (kg)*	115.5 ± 16.5 (48–182)	115.8 ± 15.9	113.4 ± 20.3	0.442
BMI [mean ± SD (range)] (kg/m^2)	42.7 ± 4.2 (17.2–61)	42.9 ± 3.9	41.3 ± 5.8	0.088
BMI > 50†	46 (6.0)	44 (6.5)	2 (2.2)	0.153
Females	647 (83.6)	568 (83.4)	79 (84.9)	0.767
Female to male ratio	5.1:1	5.0:1	5.6:1	0.767
Operative time [mean ± SD (range)] (min)	52.6 ± 19.9 (25–295)	48.9 ± 11.8	79.7 ± 38.1	<0.001
Length of stay [mean ± SD (range)] (d)	1.6 ± 0.9 (2.0) (1–9)	1.6 ± 0.9 (2.0)	1.7 ± 1.2 (2.0)	0.248
AMPs				
Dyslipidemia	118 (15.2)	104 (15.3)	14 (15.1)	>0.999
Hypertension	100 (12.9)	91 (13.4)	9 (9.7)	0.410
T2DM	111 (14.3)	103 (15.1)	8 (8.6)	0.114
OSA	67 (8.7)	62 (9.1)	5 (5.4)	0.324
Fatty liver disease	471 (60.9)	424 (62.3)	47 (50.5)	0.032
Procedures during OAGB	139 (17.9)	80 (11.7)	59 (63.4)	<0.001
Laparoscopic cholecystectomy	42 (5.4)	36 (5.3)	6 (6.5)	0.625
Laparoscopic hiatal hernia repair	75 (9.7)	44 (6.5)	31 (33.3)	<0.001
Laparoscopic gastric band removal	22 (2.8)	0 (0.0)	22 (23.6)	<0.001
Rehospitalization rate	70 (9.1)	53 (7.8)	17 (18.3)	0.003
1	47 (6.1)	35 (5.1)	12 (12.9)	0.008
2	10 (1.3)	8 (1.2)	2 (2.2)	0.343
3	7 (0.9)	6 (0.9)	1 (1.1)	0.593
4	3 (0.4)	2 (0.3)	1 (1.1)	0.120
5	1 (0.1)	0 (0.0)	1 (1.1)	0.120
7	2 (0.3)	2 (0.3)	0 (0.0)	>0.999
Reoperation rate	0 (0.0)	1 (0.15)	0 (0.0)	0.120
Death	0 (0.0)	0 (0.0)	0 (0.0)	>0.999

Table 3.
Patient data and demographic characteristics.

3. Abbreviations

a. AMP: Associated Medical Problem (comorbidity)

b. BMI: Body Mass Index

c. OAGB: One-Anastomosis Gastric Bypass

d. OSA: Obstructive Sleep Apnea

e. T2DM: Type 2 Diabetes Mellitus

4. Summary:

5. The passage outlines the data discrepancies between primary and revisional OAGB procedures and explains the statistical methods used for comparison, helping readers interpret the results accurately.

14.6 Primary vs. revisional procedures

- *Primary procedures: 88% (681 patients) were primary OAGB surgeries.*
- *Revisional procedures: 12% (93 patients) were conversions from prior surgeries, such as:*
    - *46.2% from Laparoscopic Sleeve Gastrectomy (LSG)*
    - *34.4% from Laparoscopic Adjustable Gastric Banding (LAGB)*
    - *7.5% from multiple LAGB attempts*
    - *9.6% from combined LAGB and LSG*
    - *2.2% from intragastric balloon placement* (**Table 4**)

No primary OAGB was converted to open surgery.

14.7 Operative time

Average operative time: 52.6 minutes (range: 25–295 minutes).
2020: Operative time increased to 61.3 minutes due to 32 diaphragmatic hernia repairs performed that year.

Previous bariatric procedure	Revisional OAGB (N = 93) [n (%)]
LSG	43 (46.2)
LAGB	32 (34.4)
LAGB × 2	7 (7.5)
LAGB + LSG	9 (9.6)
Intragastric balloon	2 (2.2)

LAGB indicates laparoscopic adjustable gastric banding; LSG, laparoscopic sleeve gastrectomy; OAGB, one-anastomosis gastric bypass.

Table 4.
Bariatric procedures before revisional OAGB.

Primary vs. revisional: Primary procedures took 48.9 minutes, while revisional surgeries took 79.7 minutes due to increased complexity.

Length of Stay (LOS).

Average LOS: 1.6 days (range: 1–9 days).

No significant difference in LOS between primary (1.6 days) and revisional (1.7 days) surgeries.

In summary, the majority of procedures were primary OAGBs, with revisional surgeries being conversions from previous bariatric procedures. Operative time was longer for revisional cases and influenced by combined procedures like hernia repairs, but the hospital stay was similar for both types of surgeries.

15. Comorbidities (preoperative conditions)

- *Dyslipidemia: 118 patients (15.2%) had abnormal blood lipid levels, such as high cholesterol.*
- *Hypertension: 100 patients (12.9%) had high blood pressure.*
- *Type 2 diabetes: 111 patients (14.3%) had type 2 diabetes, affecting blood sugar regulation.*
- *Obstructive sleep apnea: 67 patients (8.7%) had obstructive sleep apnea, characterized by breathing pauses during sleep.*
- *Fatty liver disease: 471 patients (60.9%) had fatty liver, indicating fat accumulation in the liver.*
- *These comorbidities can affect treatment choices, surgical risks, and postoperative recovery.*
- *Additional procedures*
- *Overall: 139 patients (17.9%) had additional surgeries along with the primary procedure.*
- *Types of additional procedures:*
- *Cholecystectomy (gallbladder removal): 42 patients (5.4%)*
- *Diaphragmatic hernia repair: 75 patients (9.7%)*
- *Gastric band removal: 22 patients (2.8%)*
- *Incisional hernia repair: 1 patient (0.1%)*
- *Adrenalectomy (adrenal gland removal): 1 patient (0.1%)*

1. Wedge resection of stomach lesion: 1 patient (0.1%)

Overall, the Mini Gastric Bypass (MGB) is very safe initially and in the long term. It has reliable weight loss and complications similar to other forms of gastric bypass [23].

DOI: http://dx.doi.org/10.5772/intechopen.1010915

16. Operative technique and key steps

16.1 The OAGB surgical procedure follows a standardized approach to ensure safety and effectiveness

Preoperative measures: Prophylactic antibiotics and sequential compression devices are administered to prevent infection and deep vein thrombosis.

Patient positioning: The patient is placed in a supine, split-leg, Trendelenburg position, which improves abdominal organ visualization. The hips are flexed for better access.

Surgical team positioning: The surgeon stands between the patient's legs, and the camera assistant is positioned on the right side. The video monitor is placed at the patient's head.

Initial access: A Veress needle is used to create pneumoperitoneum (insufflation with carbon dioxide) to a pressure of 15 mm Hg.

Port placement: A 5-port technique is used, with specific trocar placements crucial for the procedure.

Gastric decompression: A 34-Fr gastric lavage tube is inserted to remove stomach contents, aiding in better visualization. The Argyle Edlich Gastric Lavage Trays (Medtronic) are used.

In summary, this passage outlines the key setup steps for a laparoscopic procedure, focusing on patient and team positioning, creation of pneumoperitoneum, and gastric decompression to ensure the procedure is safe and effective (**Figure 2**).

The image provides a diagram showcasing the placement of trocars along with their specifications, including size and location.

- *A (5 mm)*: High epigastric on the midline.
- *B (12 mm)*: Right upper quadrant.
- *C (12 mm)*: Midline, midway between the umbilicus and the xiphoid process.
- *D (12 mm)*: Lateral on the Left upper quadrant.

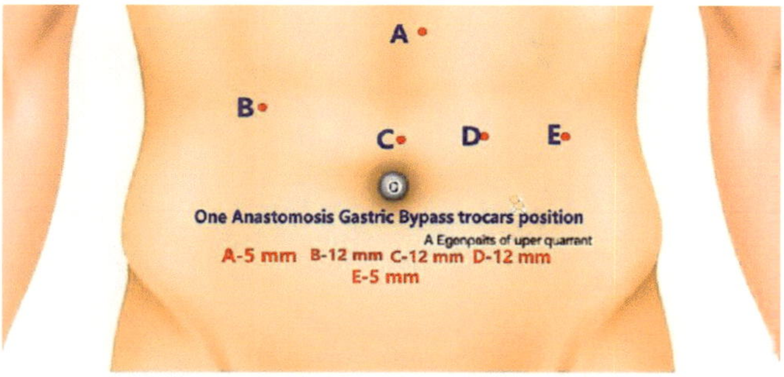

Figure 2.
The image provides a diagram showcasing the placement of trocars along with their specifications, including size and location. A (5mm): High epigastric on the midline. B (12mm): Right upper quadrant. C (12mm): Midline, midway between the umbilicus and the xiphoid process. D (12mm): Lateral on the Left upper quadrant. E (5mm): Left upper quadrant.

- *E (5 mm)*: Left upper quadrant.

16.2 Creation of the gastric pouch

Lesser sac entry: A small "window" was created between the lesser omentum and the lesser curvature of the stomach, allowing access to the lesser sac. This entry was 2 cm below the angular incisure (**Figure 3** likely illustrates this step).

Stapling: The stomach was divided using a 45 mm linear stapler. The staplers used were:

1. Ethicon Echelon Flex GST System (white cartridge)
2. Medtronic Endo GIA Tri-Staple (tan cartridge)

Stapler placement: The stapler was placed horizontally under the "crow's foot" at a right angle to the lesser curvature (**Figures 4** and **5** likely show stapler positioning and stomach division).

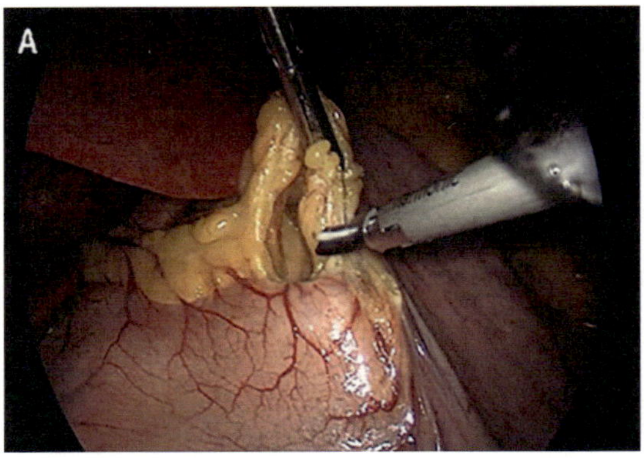

Figure 3.
Lesser Sac Entry: A small "window" was created between the lesser omentum and the lesser curvature of the stomach, allowing access to the lesser sac. This entry was 2 cm below the angular incisure (A).

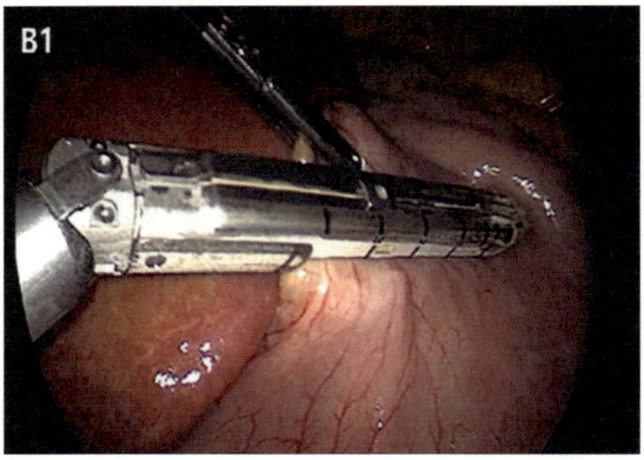

Figure 4.
Stapling: The stomach was divided using a 45 mm linear stapler. The staplers used were: a) Ethicon Echelon Flex GST System (white cartridge) b) Medtronic Endo GIA Tri-Staple (tan cartridge). Stapler Placement: The stapler was placed horizontally under the "crow's foot" at a right angle to the lesser curvature (B1).

Stomach division: The stomach was divided parallel to the lesser curvature, a critical step for pouch formation.

Pouch formation: A 34-Fr gastric lavage tube was used to guide the pouch's diameter. The pouch was sealed with 5–6 lines of 60 mm staples, directed toward the angle of His (**Figures 6** and 7 illustrate stapling completion).

- Video resources:

Video 1 - https://vimeo.com/1047470496?share=copy#t=0

Video 2 - https://vimeo.com/1047472802?share=copy#t=0

This procedure ensures the stomach is divided precisely and the pouch is formed with the appropriate size and sealing.

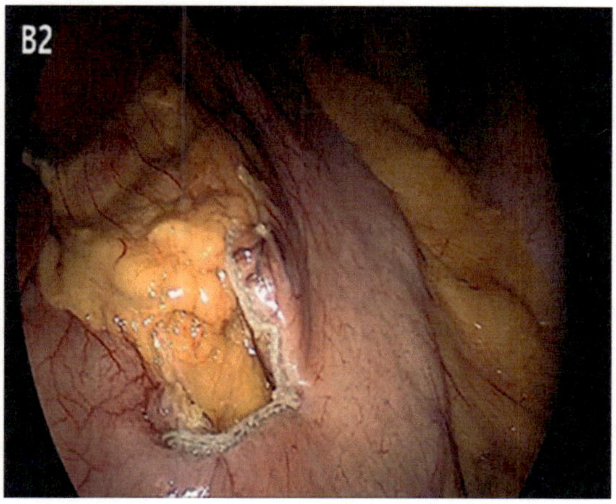

Figure 5.
Stomach Division: The stomach was divided parallel to the lesser curvature, a critical step for pouch formation (B2).

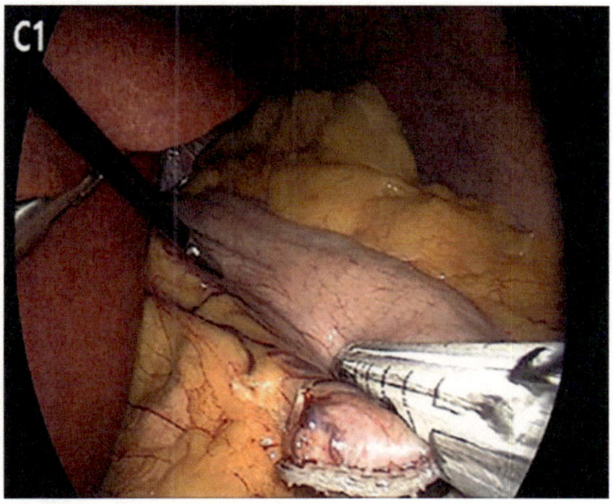

Figure 6.
Pouch Formation: A 34-Fr gastric lavage tube was used to guide the pouch's diameter. The pouch was sealed with 5 to 6 lines of 60 mm staples, directed toward the angle of His (C1).

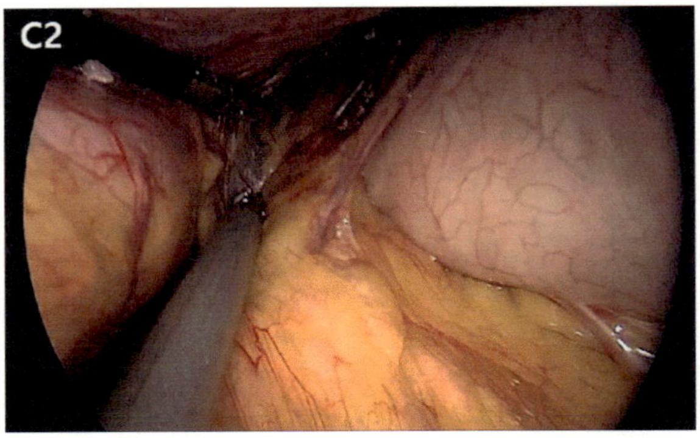

Figure 7.
Dissection of Angle of His: The angle of His, where the esophagus joins the stomach, was dissected and opened from the front (C2).

16.3 Dissection and angle of his

Dissection of angle of His: The angle of His, where the esophagus joins the stomach, was dissected and opened from the front (**Figure 8**).

Posterior access: This dissection was performed from behind the stomach (**Figure 9**).

Window creation: The process created a "window" allowing visualization of the entire left crus of the diaphragm, which plays a role in breathing (**Figure 9** illustrates this step).

In simpler terms, the surgeon separated tissues near the angle of His from behind the stomach to create an opening that provided a clear view of the diaphragm's left crus. This step is crucial for positioning the gastric pouch and preventing injury to surrounding structures, such as the oesophagus, spleen, and major blood vessels.

Anterior dissection, posterior approach: The dissection and opening of the angle of His are performed from the anterior (front) side, but the surgeon accesses this area by working posterior (behind) the stomach.

Dissection and access: The angle of His is opened from the front, but the surgeon accesses it by working behind the stomach. This involves separating tissues and structures to reach the area.

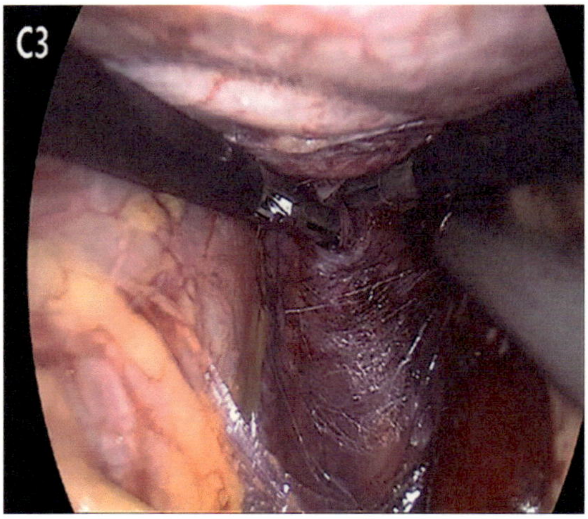

Figure 8.
Posterior Access: This dissection was performed from behind the stomach (C3).

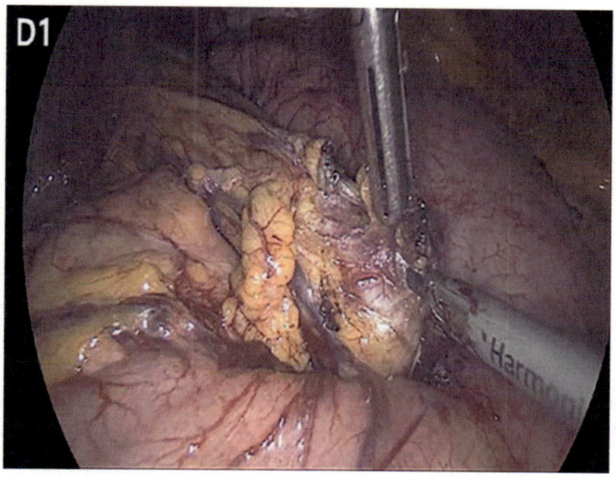

Figure 9.
The orientation of the pouch is checked to ensure it is not twisted before opening it in preparation for the anastomosis with the jejunum.

Window creation and diaphragm visualization: The dissection creates a "window" that allows the surgeon to clearly visualize the entire left crus of the diaphragm, which aids in breathing (**Figure 9** shows this step).

In simpler terms, the surgeon works behind the stomach to expose the left side of the diaphragm, which is crucial for the next steps in the procedure (Video 3 and **Figure 9** provide further details.)

Video 3 - https://vimeo.com/1047474298?share=copy#t=0

Video 4 - https://vimeo.com/1047477122?share=copy#t=0

16.4 Final stapling and pouch formation

- *Final stapling: The gastric pouch is completed by firing one or two 60-mm stapler cartridges vertically.*
- *Direction and path: Staples are directed through the "window" created earlier near the angle of His and left crus to complete pouch separation.*
- *Pouch characteristics: The narrow, long shape of the pouch is emphasized for effective volume restriction (**Figure 3** highlights this).*
- *Vessel preservation: No short gastric vessels are divided, ensuring proper blood supply and preventing complications (**Figure 7** highlights this).*

In summary, the final stapling forms the gastric pouch, with a focus on shape and preserving vessels for optimal outcomes.

Creation of the Gastro-jejunostomy (GJA)

- *GJA initiation: The creation of the GJA, the connection between the stomach pouch and the jejunum (part of the small intestine), was started.*
- *Pouch opening: A small opening was made in the lower right corner of the gastric pouch, which will be the site of the anastomosis.*

- *Stretching: This opening was stretched to prepare it for a secure connection with the jejunum.*

*In simpler terms, the surgeon made and widened an opening in the gastric pouch to initiate the connection with the small intestine, forming the GJA essential for the OAGB procedure (***Figure 10***).*

Video 5 - https://vimeo.com/1047482273?share=copy#t=0

17. Omentum retraction and bypass creation

Omentum retraction: The greater omentum was moved medially to reveal the ligament of Treitz, which marks the division between the duodenum and jejunum.

Bypass length measurement: The length of the small bowel to be bypassed was measured from the ligament of Treitz, crucial for determining the degree of malabsorption.

Jejunal loop elevation: A loop of jejunum was lifted antecolic (in front of the colon), rotated clockwise, and brought up to the gastric pouch.

Anastomosis: The jejunum was connected to the lower right end of the gastric pouch with a 45 mm linear stapler.

Bypass length: The anastomosis point was about 150–200 cm downstream from the ligament of Treitz, determining the length of the bypassed jejunum.

In simpler terms, the surgeon identified a key intestinal landmark, measured the jejunum to bypass, elevated and positioned it, and stapled it to the gastric pouch, with the bypass length impacting nutrient absorption (**Figure 11**).

(**Figures 12** and **13**). Video 6 - https://vimeo.com/1047483338?share=copy#t=0

17.1 Bile-pancreatic loop (BPL) length and adjustments

BPL length variation: The bile-pancreatic loop (BPL), carrying bile and pancreatic secretions but not food, typically ranges from 150 to 250 cm, with a standard length of 180 cm.

Adjustment factors: BPL length is customized based on the patient's preoperative BMI and the surgeon's judgment.

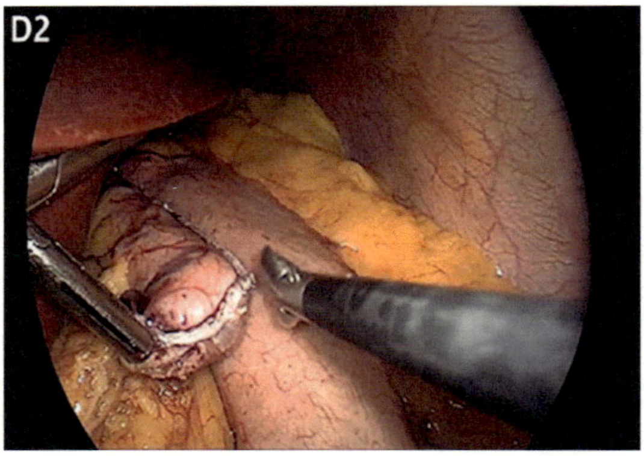

Figure 10.
Pouch Opening: A small opening was made in the lower right corner of the gastric pouch, which will be the site of the anastomosis. This opening was stretched to prepare it for a secure anastomosis with the jejunum.

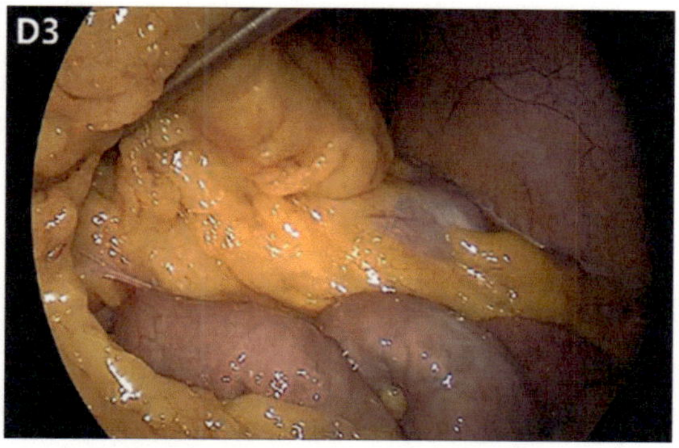

Figure 11.
Omentum Retraction: The greater omentum was moved medially to reveal the ligament of Treitz, which marks the division between the duodenum and jejunum (D3).

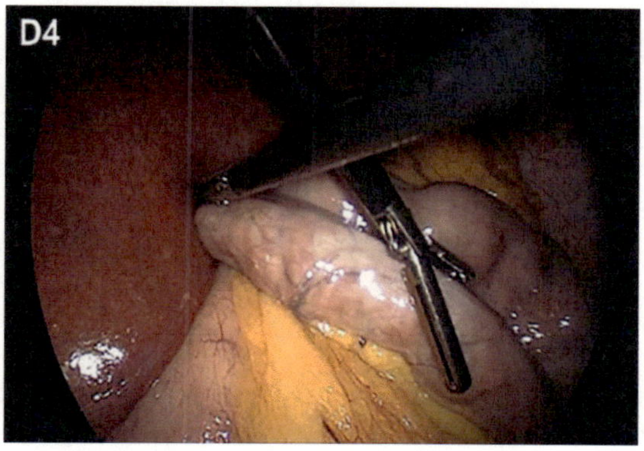

Figure 12.
Bypass Length Measurement: The length of the small bowel to be bypassed was measured from the ligament of Treitz, crucial for determining the degree of malabsorption (D4).

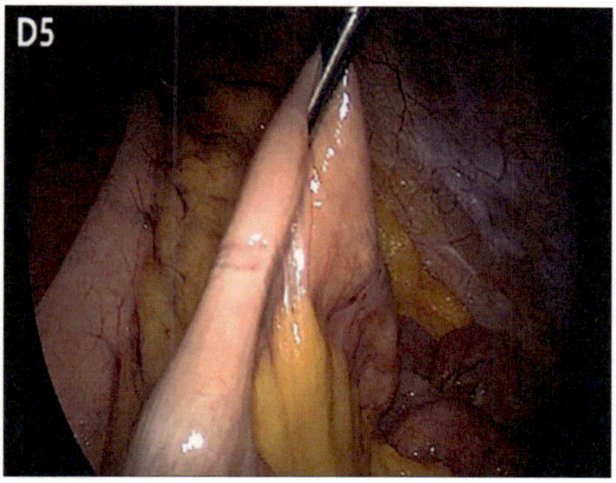

Figure 13.
Jejunal Loop Elevation: A loop of jejunum was lifted antecolic (in front of the colon), rotated clockwise, and brought up to the gastric pouch (D5).

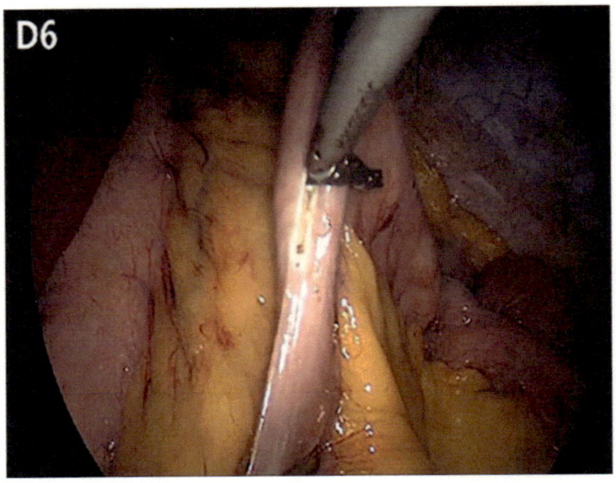

Figure 14.
Enterotomy Location: An enterotomy is made 150 to 200 cm distal from the ligament of Treitz (D6).

Enterotomy location: An enterotomy is made 150–200 cm distal from the ligament of Treitz (**Figure 14**).

BMI and revisional surgery: Patients with a BMI >50 kg/m^2 or undergoing revisional surgery for weight regain typically have a longer BPL (200–250 cm).

Debate on optimal length: The ideal BPL length for both primary and revisional OAGB remains a topic of debate within the surgical community.

Importance of total small bowel measurement: Measuring the entire small bowel is crucial to ensure enough remains in the "food stream" after the anastomosis.

Revisional surgery considerations: BPL length is particularly significant in revisional surgeries.

In summary, the BPL length is key to the OAGB procedure, with adjustments made based on factors like BMI and whether the surgery is primary or revisional. Accurate measurement of the total small bowel is crucial for optimal function after surgery.

Video 6 - https://vimeo.com/1047483338?share=copy#t=0

18. Distal pouch anastomosis

Anastomosis: The distal end of the gastric pouch was connected to the side of the small bowel using a 45 mm linear stapler.

Simplified: The surgeon used staples to join the bottom of the stomach pouch to the small intestine, allowing food to pass into the bypassed portion of the small bowel (**Figure 15**).

(**Figure 15**). Video 6 - https://vimeo.com/1047483338?share=copy#t=0

A 3–4 cm anastomosis was created posteriorly (**Figures 16** and **17**).

Video 7 - https://vimeo.com/1047485996?share=copy#t=0

18.1 Limb placement

- *Afferent limb:* Positioned on the patient's left side (leading to the stomach pouch).
- *Efferent limb:* Positioned on the patient's right side (leading away from the pouch).

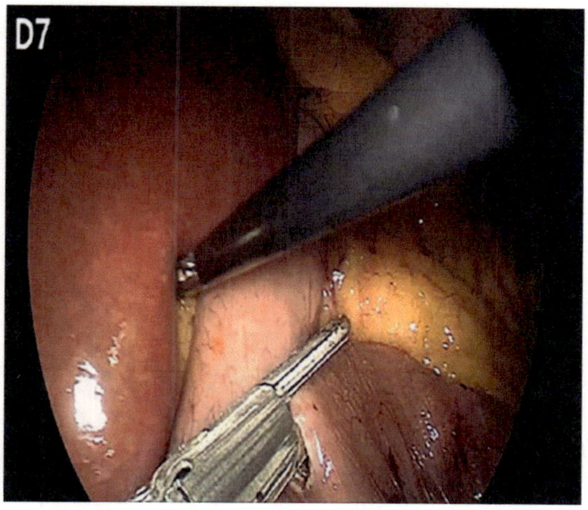

Figure 15.
Anastomosis: The distal end of the gastric pouch was connected to the side of the small bowel using a 45 mm linear stapler. Simplified: The surgeon used staples to join the bottom of the stomach pouch to the small intestine, allowing food to pass into the bypassed portion of the small bowel (D7).

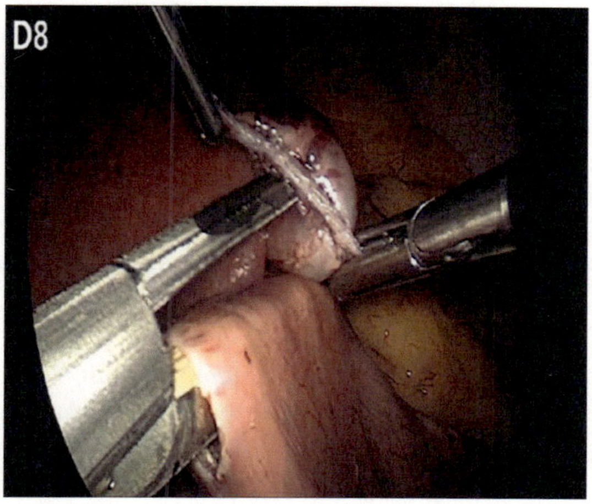

Figure 16.
A 3- to 4-cm anastomosis was created posteriorly (D8, D9).

- *Reason:* Proper placement prevents torsion (twisting) of the intestinal mesentery, ensuring blood flow and reducing complications.

In short, the correct positioning of the limbs is crucial to avoid twisting and ensure adequate blood supply.

- A *34-Fr gastric lavage tube* was passed through the anastomosis into the efferent limb.

- *Calibration:* The tube served as a guide to ensure the anastomosis had the correct diameter, preventing it from being too narrow and ensuring proper food passage.

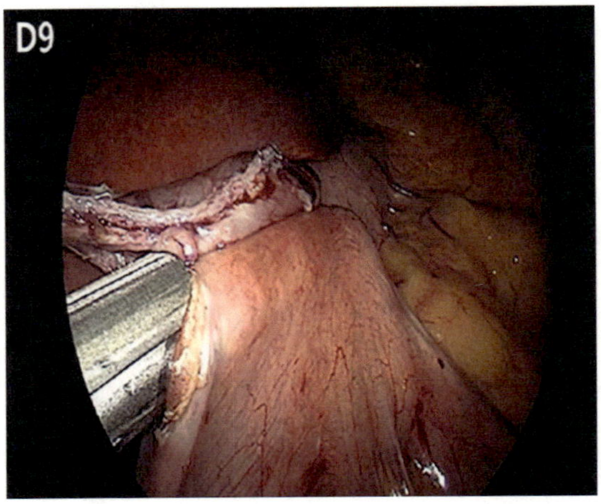

Figure 17.
Anastomosis: The distal end of the gastric pouch was connected to the side of the small bowel using a 45 mm linear stapler (D9).

- A tube was inserted through the connection between the stomach and intestine to make sure the opening was the right size. This step helps prevent future complications related to a too-small anastomosis (**Figure 18**).

In short, the tube was used to ensure the anastomosis was the right size to prevent future complications.

18.2 Stapler hole closure

- *Suture type:* A *3/0 VLoc* barbed absorbable suture was used to close the stapler holes.

- *Technique:* The suture was placed in a *continuous, running* fashion through the seromuscular-seromuscular layers of the stomach and intestine.

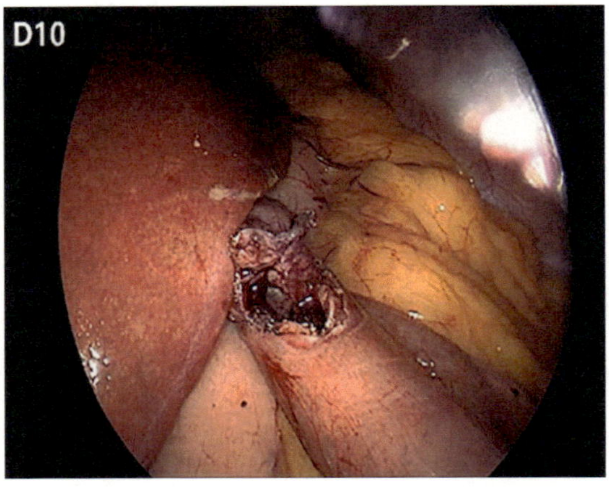

Figure 18.
A tube was inserted through the connection between the stomach and intestine to make sure the opening was the right size. This step helps prevent future complications related to a too-small anastomosis (D10).

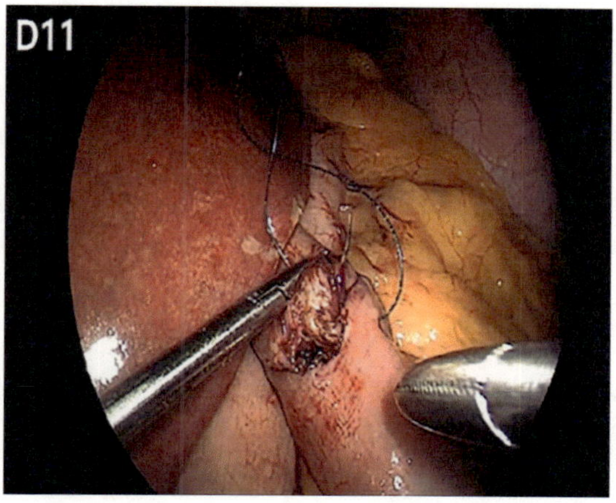

Figure 19.
Suture Type: A 3/0 VLoc barbed absorbable suture was used to close the stapler holes. Technique: The suture was placed in a continuous, running fashion through the seromuscular-seromuscular layers of the stomach and intestine. Invagination: The suture helped turn the proximal staple line inward, ensuring a smoother connection and reducing leak risks (D11).

- *Invagination:* The suture helped turn the proximal staple line inward, ensuring a smoother connection and reducing leak risks.

In short, the surgeon used a special suture to reinforce the connection between the stomach and intestine, ensuring a secure, leak-free *end-to-side gastrojejunostomy (GJA).* (**Figure 19**) Video 8 - https://vimeo.com/1047489632?share=copy#t=0
Video 8 - https://vimeo.com/1047489632?share=copy#t=0
Video 9 - https://vimeo.com/1047490633?share=copy#t=0

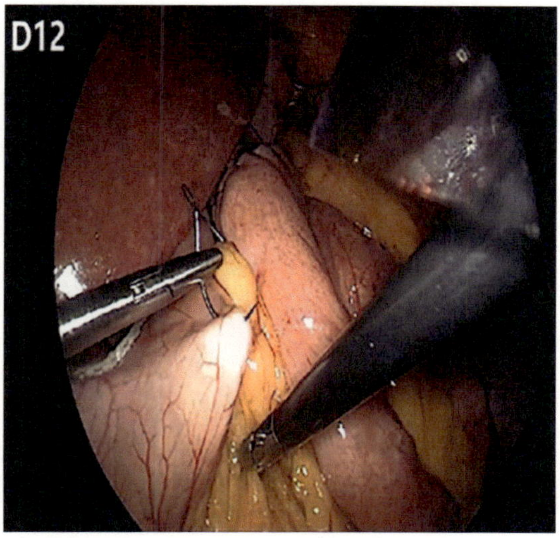

Figure 20.
Loop Fixation: The efferent loop (food-carrying limb) was attached to the bypassed stomach while the afferent loop (digestive fluid-carrying limb) was secured to the gastric pouch (Figures D14, D15). Isoperistaltic Conduit: The afferent limb was positioned higher than the efferent loop, ensuring that peristalsis moves food and digestive juices in the same direction (D12).

18.3 Loop fixation and isoperistaltic conduit

Loop fixation: The efferent loop (food-carrying limb) was attached to the bypassed stomach, while the afferent loop (digestive fluid-carrying limb) was secured to the gastric pouch (**Figures 20** and **21**).

Isoperistaltic conduit: The afferent limb was positioned higher than the efferent loop, ensuring that peristalsis moves food and digestive juices in the same direction (**Figure 22**).

18.4 Gastrojejunostomy testing

- *Leak test:* Methylene blue dye was introduced via a *34-Fr gastric lavage tube* to check for leaks at the *GJA* (**Figure 23**).

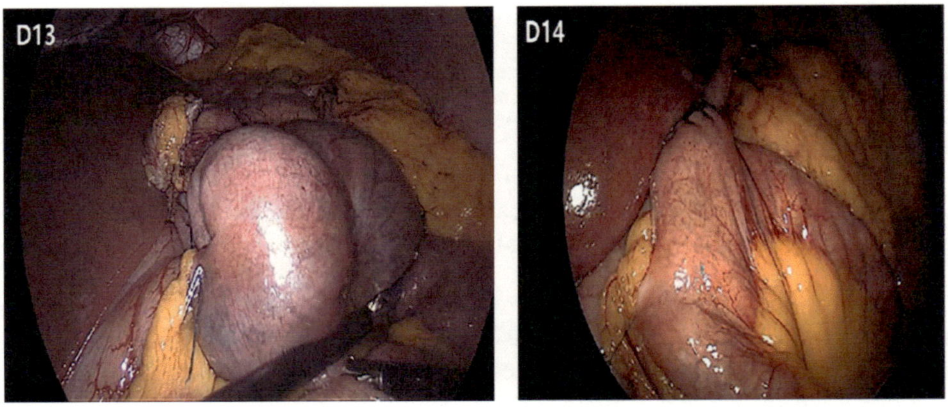

Figure 21.
Leak Test: Methylene blue dye was introduced via a 34-Fr gastric lavage tube to check for leaks at the GJA (D13). Loop Fixation: The efferent loop (food-carrying limb) was attached to the bypassed stomach, while the afferent loop (digestive fluid-carrying limb) was secured to the gastric pouch (D14).

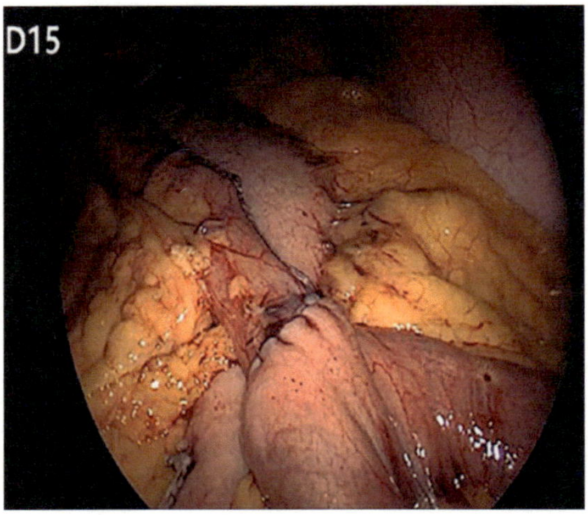

Figure 22.
Limb Placement, Afferent Limb: Positioned on the patient's left side (leading to the stomach pouch). Efferent Limb: Positioned on the patient's right side (leading away from the pouch). Reason: Proper placement prevents torsion (twisting) of the intestinal mesentery, ensuring blood flow and reducing complications (D15).

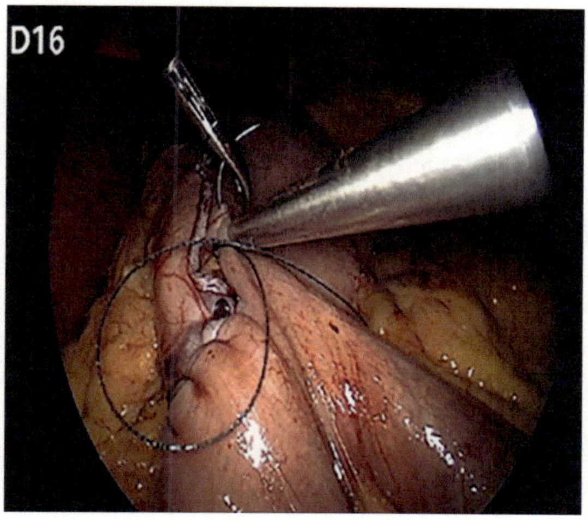

Figure 23.
A single absorbable suture was placed, attaching the afferent limb to the left side of the gastric pouch, 3 cm proximal to the GJA (D16).

- *Tubes and drains:* Routine *nasogastric tubes and surgical drains were not used* postoperatively.

Video 10 - https://vimeo.com/1047492295?share=copy#t=0

18.5 Anti-reflux suture

A single *absorbable suture* was placed, attaching the *afferent limb* to the left side of the gastric pouch, *3 cm proximal to the GJA* (Figure D16).

Purpose: To *facilitate bile flow* toward the efferent limb and prevent reflux into the gastric pouch.

In summary, the passage describes how the surgical team tested the connection between the stomach and intestine for leaks, notes their practice of not routinely using certain tubes and drains, and explains the placement of a suture to help prevent reflux of digestive juices (**Figure 16**).

18.6 Standardization and learning curve

The learning curve, as described by Ebbinghaus in 1885, is fundamental in surgical proficiency [24]. In OAGB, repeated procedures facilitated technical refinements, leading to a standardized surgical approach. [25, 26]. This standardization, implemented between 2016 and 2021, correlated with decreased operative times, shorter hospital stays, reduced morbidity, and an increased patient volume, rising from 66 patients in 2016 to 191 in 2021. The mean operative time in this study was 48.9 minutes for primary procedures and 52.6 minutes for the combined group, with a mean length of stay (LOS) of 1.6 days. These metrics compare favorably with published data, which report mean operative times of 37.5 minutes in a large series and 73.5 minutes in a systematic review, and LOS ranging from 1 to 5 days.

18.7 Early complications

Early complications, occurring within 30 days post-surgery, include leaks, bleeding, and strictures. The overall complication rate typically ranges from 3.5 to 7.9%. The International Federation for the Surgery of Obesity and Metabolic Disorders (IFSO) reported a 5.51% early complication rate in 19,051 OAGB procedures, with a 1.01% reoperation rate. Primary procedures had a 4.91% complication rate, while revisional procedures had 7.9%. In this study, the early complication rate was 2.1%, with major complications at 0.3%, minor complications at 2.0%, and no reoperations. This is notably lower than rates reported in larger reviews, which cite a mean early complication rate of 4.7% and major complications ranging from 0 to 5.5%. The study reported no early mortality, further supporting the procedure's safety profile.

18.8 Leak prevalence and management

Leaks, the most common complication, typically occur within the first 3 days and can lead to severe sequelae. Rates range from 0.1 to 1.9%, with a systematic review of 12,807 patients reporting a 0.96% leak rate [27]. Causes include issues with closure materials, poor blood flow, and conditions affecting wound healing. Symptoms include abdominal pain, fever, and tachycardia. Diagnosis involves monitoring, physical examination, and imaging. Management includes fluid stabilization, infection control, nutritional support, and, in severe cases, surgical intervention. The leak rate in this study was 0.3%, lower than rates reported in other large studies.

18.9 Bleeding and other early complications

- *Bleeding prevalence: Bleeding is the second most common early complication; it typically originates from the gastric pouch staple line, blood vessels during dissection, or the GJA [28].*

- *Diagnosis and management: Bleeding may be intraluminal (within the digestive tract) or intra-abdominal (in the abdomen). with rates ranging from 0.9 to 1.7% [27, 29] in various studies. Most cases are managed conservatively, but a few may require surgical intervention.*

- *Current study's bleeding rate: The study observed a 0.4% postoperative bleeding rate (3 out of 774 patients), all managed conservatively without surgery.*

venous thromboembolism (VTE), with an incidence of 0.3–2.4%, and gastric remnant distension. VTE prevention involves early mobilization and low-dose unfractionated heparin or low-molecular-weight heparin (LMWH) [30].

18.10 Late complications

Late complications include nutrient deficiencies, internal hernias (IH), marginal ulcers, dumping syndrome, and bile reflux. IH occurred in 2.8% of patients, with diagnosis relying on CT scans [31]. Marginal ulcers are treated with proton pump inhibitors (PPIs) and lifestyle modifications, Surgical Options: Required in severe cases (dilatation or bypass revision) [31].

Complication	OAGB population (N = 774) [n (%)]	Treatment
Leak	2 (0.3)	(1) Percutaneous drainage, ICU stay
		(2) Re-laparoscopy with drainage
Bleeding	3 (0.4)	Conservative treatment
Wound infection	1 (0.1)	Conservative treatment
Respiratory issues*	3 (0.4)	Conservative treatment, ICU stay
Acute kidney failure	1 (0.1)	Conservative treatment
Urinary tract infection	2 (0.3)	Antibiotics
ICU stay	4 (0.5)	
Total morbidity	16 (2.1)	

**Difficult weaning off intubation, pneumothorax, hypoxia.*
ICU indicates intensive care unit; OAGB, one-anastomosis gastric bypass.

Table 5.
Early postoperative complications after OAGB.

References	No. cases	Complication rate (%)	Major complication rate (%)	Mortality rate
This study	774	2.1	0.3	0.0
Carbajo et al. [10]	1200	2.33	1.33	0.17
Wang et al. [19]	423	5.9	1.65	0.47
Chevallier et al. [28]	1000	3.5	—	0.2
Lessing et al. [29]	407	4.22	2.46	0
Musella et al. [30]	2678	3.14	0.68	0.11
Taha et al. [31]	1520	3.16	0.47	0.13
Kular et al. [32]	1054	4.65	1.33	0.19
Carbajo et al. [32]	209	3.83	1.44	0.96
Musella et al. [33]	954	5.57	2.1	0.21
Noun et al. [34]	1000	3.4	0.6	0
Kansou et al. [35]	136	6.62	4.1	0

Table 6.
Comparative individual one-anastomosis gastric bypass study complication and mortality rates.

Dumping syndrome is managed through dietary changes and medication. Bile reflux, with a reported incidence varying widely (7.8–55.5%), may necessitate conversion to Roux-en-Y Gastric Bypass (RYGB) [32, 33].

Mortality and standardization:

Overall complication rate: Within 30 days post-surgery, complication rates range from 3.5 to 7.9%, including major issues like leaks, bleeding, and strictures [29].

The International Federation for the Surgery of Obesity and Metabolic Disorders (IFSO) reported that among 19,051 one-anastomosis gastric bypass (OAGB) procedures, the early complication rate was 5.51%, with a reoperation rate of 1.01%.

Specifically, primary procedures had an early complication rate of 4.91%, while revisional procedures had a rate of 7.9% [34].

Total complication rate: Between 3.5 and 7.9% in early OAGB recovery, with 3–8 out of every 100 patients experiencing complications (**Tables 3** and 5).

Comparison to other studies: Major complications:

Large sample size: A review with 12,807 patients showed a mean early complication rate of 4.7%, with major complications ranging from 0 to 5.5% [27].

The current study's complication rates are lower than those reported in large systematic reviews and individual studies. Importantly, the study reported no early mortality, reinforcing the safety of the procedure (**Table 6**).

In summary, the current study shows low complication rates, efficient operative times, and a positive safety profile compared to other OAGB studies, particularly with its low reoperation and complication rates.

19. Revisional OAGB and conversion to RYGB

Revisional One-Anastomosis Gastric Bypass (OAGB) surgery is considered a viable option for patients experiencing failure following initial restrictive bariatric procedures. While OAGB demonstrates general safety and effectiveness, its inherent malabsorptive nature can, in some cases, lead to severe protein-energy malnutrition (PEM), potentially necessitating further surgical intervention to restore normal anatomy. A comprehensive literature review encompassing 26 studies and 1771 patients who underwent revisional OAGB/Mini Gastric Bypass (MGB) following failed restrictive surgeries revealed significant improvements. Specifically, Body Mass Index (BMI) values averaged 31.52 kg/m^2 at 1 year, 31.40 kg/m^2 at 3 years, and 30.54 kg/m^2 at 5 years post-revision. Diabetes remission rates were 65.16% at 1 year, 65.37% at 3 years, and 78.10% at 5 years. While improvements in gastroesophageal reflux disease (GERD) were noted, 7.4% of patients developed new-onset GERD post-revision. Leakage was identified as the most common major complication; however, OAGB/MGB remains a feasible and effective revisional strategy [35]

Severe bile reflux represents a recognized long-term complication following OAGB. In a cohort of 16 patients experiencing severe bile reflux post-OAGB, conversion to Roux-en-Y Gastric Bypass (RYGB) was performed. Symptom onset occurred, on average, 58.3 months post-initial OAGB. All patients presented with pain, 81.3% experienced vomiting, and 43.8% reported dysphagia. Endoscopic evaluation revealed bile presence in all patients, with 31.3% exhibiting marginal ulceration and 50% gastritis. The mean alimentary limb length at revision was 37.7 cm, ranging from 20 to 62 cm. Following an average 14.9-month post-conversion follow-up, all 16 patients reported complete resolution of bile reflux symptoms [36].

20. Conclusion

The authors of this study are trying to standardize the procedure. That makes sense because variations in surgical technique can lead to different outcomes, so having a standardized approach could improve consistency and safety. The paper probably details the steps they took to create this standardization, maybe things like the size of the gastric pouch, the location of the anastomosis, the length of the biliopancreatic limb, etc.

The technical aspects section would describe exactly how the surgery is performed. For example, how they create the gastric pouch—using staplers, how they measure the limbs, how they perform the anastomosis (hand-sewn vs. stapled), and any other specific steps taken to ensure uniformity across procedures.

The early outcomes would include things like weight loss results, complication rates (both during surgery and post-op), hospital stay length, and any adverse effects like leaks, infections, or nutritional issues. Since it is early outcomes, they are probably looking at data from the first 30 days or so after surgery, maybe up to a year.

The authors involved are from different institutions, which suggests a collaborative effort. Maybe they compared their standardized technique outcomes to previous non-standardized approaches or other procedures. I should check if they have a control group or if this is a retrospective/prospective study.

Looking at the names, Nasser Sakran and Mohamad Hamoud are known bariatric surgeons, so their involvement adds credibility. The study being in a journal like Obesity Surgery or similar would make sense. The methods section would explain the patient selection criteria, the surgical protocol, data collection methods, and statistical analysis.

Potential strengths of the study could be a large sample size, detailed technical description, and multi-center involvement. Weaknesses might be short follow-up time (since it is early outcomes), possible selection bias, or lack of long-term data on complications like nutritional deficiencies or bile reflux.

I should also consider how this study contributes to existing literature. OAGB has been controversial in some circles because of concerns about long-term complications, so a standardized technique that reduces variability might help in comparing outcomes across different studies and improving patient safety.

Wait, the term "one-anastomosis" versus "mini" gastric bypass—is OAGB the same as the mini gastric bypass? I think they are similar or the same procedure. Some surgeons prefer OAGB as the terminology now.

In the technical aspects, they might mention things like the length of the gastric pouch, starting from the angle of His, the size of the pouch, the antecolic vs. retrocolic route for the anastomosis, the length of the biliopancreatic limb (which could affect malabsorption), and the type of anastomosis (e.g., linear vs. circular stapler).

For early outcomes, they will report on operative time, conversion rates to open surgery, intraoperative complications like bleeding or organ injury, and postoperative complications such as leaks, strictures, DVT, pulmonary embolism, and mortality. Weight loss metrics like % excess weight loss at 3, 6, and 12 months might be included. Also, the resolution of comorbidities like diabetes, hypertension, and sleep apnea.

They might also discuss how their standardization affected outcomes compared to previous reports. If their complication rates are lower, that suggests standardization helps. If operative times are consistent, that is another plus.

I wonder if they addressed the learning curve for surgeons adopting this standardized technique. If they included multiple surgeons across centers, they might analyze outcomes relative to surgeon experience.

Nutritional outcomes are important too—iron, B12, and calcium levels post-op. But since it is early outcomes, maybe they only look at acute issues rather than long-term deficiencies.

Another point is patient selection. Did they use standard bariatric criteria—BMI over 40, or over 35 with comorbidities? Any exclusion criteria, like previous gastric surgery, that could affect outcomes?

In the results, they will probably have demographic data—age, gender, baseline BMI, and comorbidities. Then, surgical outcomes like operative time, length of stay, and complications. Weight loss at various intervals. Statistical tests would check for significance in differences, maybe correlations between technique variables and outcomes.

In the discussion, they will interpret the results in the context of existing literature. They might argue that their standardized technique reduces variability and improves safety, making OAGB a more viable option. They might address limitations, like the need for long-term follow-up studies.

I should also consider if there are any conflicting interests, like funding from medical device companies, but that is usually in the disclosures.

Overall, this study seems to contribute a detailed protocol for OAGB, aiming to reduce surgical variability and improve early postoperative outcomes. The findings could help other surgeons adopt OAGB with a standardized approach, potentially leading to better comparative studies in the future.

The study provides a validated, stepwise approach to OAGB, demonstrating its safety and efficacy in early outcomes. Standardization facilitates broader adoption and reliable comparison in bariatric research, positioning OAGB as a viable option for morbid obesity management. Surgeons are encouraged to adhere to detailed protocols to optimize patient outcomes.

Author details

Mohamad Hamoud
Surgery Department, Holy Family Hospital, Bar-Ilan University, Nazareth, Israel

*Address all correspondence to: dr.hamoud@gmail.com

References

[1] Emmerich SD, Fryar CD, Stierman B, Ogden CL. Obesity and Severe Obesity Prevalence in Adults: United States, August 2021–August 2022 (National Center for Health Statistics Data Brief No. 508). Hyattsville, Maryland, USA: National Center for Health Statistics; (NCHS) 2024. DOI: 10.15620/cdc/159281

[2] Dimitriadis GK, Randeva MS, Miras AD. Potential hormone mechanisms of bariatric surgery. Current Obesity Reports. 2017-09;**6**(3):253-265

[3] Sudlow A, Pournaras DJ, et al. The metabolic benefits of different bariatric operations: What procedure to choose. Endocrine Connections. 2020;**9**(2):R28-R35. DOI: 10.1530/EC-19-0467

[4] Cummings DE et al. Bariatric/metabolic surgery to treat type 2 diabetes in patients with a BMI <35 kg/m2. Diabetes Care. 2016;**39**(6):924-933. DOI: 10.2337/dc16-0350

[5] Faria GR et al. A brief history of bariatric surgery. Porto Biomedical Journal. 2017;**2**(3):90-92. DOI: 10.1016/j.pbj.2017.01.008

[6] Hopkins KD, Lehmann ED. Successful medical treatment of obesity in 10th century Spain. Lancet. 1995;**346**(8972):452. DOI: 10.1016/s0140-6736(95)92830-8

[7] Kremen AJ, Linner JH, Nelson CH. An experimental evaluation of the nutritional importance of proximal and distal small intestine. Annals of Surgery. 1954;**140**(3):439-448. DOI: 10.1097/00000658-195409000-00018 Ann Surg. Obesity Surgery 29(14) DOI: 10.1007/s11695-019-04018-9

[8] Rodriguez J, Patrick O'Leary J. History of the development of metabolic/bariatric surgery. In: The ASMBS Textbook of Bariatric Surgery. 2nd ed. Springer. pp. 37-46. DOI: 10.1007/978-3-030-27021-6_3

[9] Organization for Economic Co-Operation and Development (OECD). Obesity Update. 2012. Available from: https://www.oecd.org/health/49716427.pdf [Accessed: June 16, 2022]

[10] Parikh M, Eisenberg D, Johnson J, et al. American Society for metabolic and bariatric surgery review of the literature on one anastomosis gastric bypass. Surgery for Obesity and Related Diseases. 2018;**14**:1088-1092. Current Obesity Reports 2017;6(3):253-265. doi:10.1007/s13679-017-0276-5

[11] Howard R, Chao GF, Yang J, Thumma J, Chhabra K, Arterburn DE, et al. Comparative safety of sleeve gastrectomy and gastric bypass up to 5 years after surgery in patients with severe obesity. JAMA Surgery. 2021;**156**(12):1160-1169. DOI: 10.1001/jamasurg.2021.4981

[12] Homan J, Betzel B, Aarts EO, Dogan K, van Laarhoven KJ, Janssen IM, et al. Vitamin and mineral deficiencies after biliopancreatic diversion and biliopancreatic diversion with duodenal switch--the rule rather than the exception. Obesity Surgery. 2015;**25**(9):1626-1632. DOI: 10.1007/s11695-015-1570-5

[13] Dai Y, Luo B, Li W. Incidence and risk factors for cholelithiasis after bariatric surgery: A systematic review and meta-analysis. Lipids in Health and Disease. 2023;**22**(1):5. DOI: 10.1186/s12944-023-01774-7

[14] Spinos D, Skarentzos K, Esagian SM, Seymour KA, Economopoulos KP. The effectiveness of single-anastomosis Duodenoileal bypass with sleeve gastrectomy/one anastomosis duodenal switch (SADI-S/OADS): An updated systematic review. Obesity Surgery. 2021;**31**(4):1790-1800. DOI: 10.1007/s11695-020-05188-7. Epub 2021 Jan 16

[15] ugerman HJ, Wolfe LG, Sica DA, Clore JN. Diabetes and hypertension in severe obesity and effects of gastric bypass-induced weight loss. Annals of Surgery. 2003;**237**(6):751-756; discussion 757-8. DOI: 10.1097/01.SLA.0000071560.76194.11

[16] Rutledge R. The mini-gastric bypass: Experience with the first 1,274 cases. Obesity Surgery. 2001;**11**(3):276-280. DOI: 10.1381/096089201321056161

[17] Mahawar KK, Jennings N, Brown J, et al. "Mini" gastric bypass: Systematic review of a controversial procedure. Obesity Surgery. 2013;**23**(12):1890-1898. DOI: 10.1007/s11695-013-1000-0

[18] Castaneda D et al. Risk of suicide and self-harm is increased after bariatric surgery-a systematic review and meta-analysis. Obesity Surgery. 2019;**29**(1):322-333. DOI: 10.1007/s11695-018-3493-4

[19] Neovius M et al. Bariatric surgery & suicide: Results from two controlled matched cohort studies. The Lancet Diabetes and Endocrinology. 2018;**6**(3):197-207. DOI: 10.1016/S2213-8587(17)30437-0

[20] Sakran N, Hamoud M, et al. Standardization of the one-anastomosis gastric bypass procedure for morbid obesity: Technical aspects and early outcomes. Surgical Laparoscopy, Endoscopy and Percutaneous Techniques. 2023;**33**(2):162-170. DOI: 10.1097/SLE.0000000000001148

[21] Conceição EM et al. Eating disorders and problematic eating behaviors before and after bariatric surgery: Characterization, assessment, and association with treatment outcomes. European Eating Disorders Review. 2015;**23**(6):455-464. DOI: 10.1002/erv.2403

[22] Conceiao EM, Goldschmidt AB. Psychopathology and weight regain after bariatric surgery: A systematic review and meta-analysis. Obesity Reviews. 2019;**20**(1):12-26. Eur Eat Disord Rev. 2015;23(6):417-425. doi: 10.1002/erv.2397

[23] Rutledge R, Walsh TR. Continued excellent results with the mini-gastric bypass: Six-year study in 2,410 patients. Obesity Surgery. 2005;**15**(10):1304-1308. DOI: 10.1381/096089205775381206

[24] Ebbinghaus H. Memory: A Contribution to Experimental Psychology. Dover Publications; 1885

[25] Lo HC. The learning curve of one anastomosis gastric bypass and its impact as a preceding procedure to roux-en-Y gastric bypass: Initial experience of one hundred and five consecutive cases. BMC Surgery. 2020;**20**:37. DOI: 10.1186/s12893-020-00714-2

[26] Wehrtmann FS, de la Garza JR, Kowalewski KF, et al. Learning curves of laparoscopic roux-en-Y gastric bypass and sleeve gastrectomy in bariatric surgery: A systematic review and introduction of a standardization. Obesity Surgery. 2020;**30**(2):640-656. DOI: 10.1007/s11695-019-04294-x

[27] Armar CD, Mahawar KK. One anastomosis (mini) gastric bypass is now an established bariatric procedure: A systematic review of 12,807 patients.

Obesity Surgery. 2018;**28**(9):2956-2967. DOI: 10.1007/s11695-018-3327-0

[28] Chevallier JM, Arman GA, Guenzi M, et al. One thousand single anastomosis (omega loop) gastric bypasses to treat morbid obesity in a 7-year period: Outcomes show few complications. Obesity Surgery. 2015;**25**(11):2027-2033. DOI: 10.1007/s11695-015-1674-

[29] Sakran N, Sherf-Dagan S, Hod K, Kaplan U, Azaria B, Raziel A. Assuta bariatric surgeons collaborative. One anastomosis gastric bypass in 6722 patients: Early outcomes from a private hospital registry. Journal of Clinical Medicine. 2023;**12**(21):6872. DOI: 10.3390/jcm12216872

[30] Carvalho L, Almeida RF, Nora M, Guimarães M. Thromboembolic complications after bariatric surgery: Is the high risk real? Cureus. 2023;**15**(1):e33444. DOI: 10.7759/cureus.33444

[31] Petruccian N. Internal hernia after one anastomosis gastric bypass (OAGB): Lessons learned from a retrospective series of 3368 consecutive patients undergoing OAGB with a biliopancreatic limb of 150cm. Obesity Surgery. 2021;**31**(6):2537-2544. DOI: 10.1007/s11695-021-05269-1

[32] Csendes A. Bile reflux after one anastomosis gastric bypass. Obesity Surgery. 2020;**30**(7). DOI: 10.1007/s11695-020-04567-4

[33] Ferrer-Márquez M et al. Bile reflux and marginal ulcers after one-anastomosis gastric bypass (OAGB). A Narrative Review Cirugía Española (English Edition). 2023;**101**(Supplement 4):S69-S75

[34] De Luca M, Piatto G, Merola G, et al. IFSO update position statement on one anastomosis gastric bypass (OAGB). Obesity Surgery. 2021;**31**:3251-3278. DOI: 10.1007/s11695-021-05413-x

[35] Kermansaravi M, Shahmiri SS, Davarpanah Jazi AH, Valizadeh R, Berardi G, Vitiello A, et al. One anastomosis/mini-gastric bypass (OAGB/MGB) as revisional surgery following primary restrictive bariatric procedures: A systematic review and meta-analysis. Obesity Surgery. 2021;**31**(1):370-383. DOI: 10.1007/s11695-020-05079-x. Epub 2020 Oct 28

[36] Swartz DE, Mobley E, Felix EL. Bile reflux after roux-en-Y gastric bypass: An unrecognized cause of postoperative pain. Surgery for Obesity and Related Diseases. 2009;**5**(1):27-30. DOI: 10.1016/j.soard.2008.10.009. Epub 2008 Oct 30

Chapter 7

Body Contouring and Metabolic Improvement Updates and Perspectives: VASER Liposuction and Ketogenic Diet for BMI above 35

Hasan Ali

Abstract

This chapter presents a multidisciplinary approach to obesity management by integrating VASER liposuction and a ketogenic diet, specifically targeting patients with a BMI above 35. Obesity treatments often fail to achieve dual objectives: substantial weight reduction and effective body contouring, particularly when post-weight loss skin laxity is a concern. VASER liposuction, a minimally invasive technique, addresses these challenges by promoting precise fat removal and superior skin tightening through collagen remodeling, and contouring improvements. Paired with the ketogenic diet, which induces ketosis to optimize fat metabolism, reduce systemic inflammation, and improve insulin sensitivity, this approach bridges gaps in traditional obesity management. A comprehensive analysis of a case series demonstrates the efficacy of this combined strategy, highlighting metabolic benefits such as improved lipid profiles, cardiovascular health, and hormonal balance alongside esthetic enhancements. Notably, several patients achieved significant weight and BMI reductions even without combining VASER liposuction with dietary interventions, underscoring the standalone potential of the procedure for lower BMI individuals. Patient satisfaction ratings averaged 8.5 out of 10, reflecting the dual efficacy of esthetic and metabolic improvements. Key topics such as patient selection, procedural techniques, postoperative care, and long-term outcomes are discussed. This innovative approach offers a transformative alternative to conventional methods, providing sustainable results and addressing the multifaceted challenges of obesity. The findings emphasize the relevance of integrating advanced technologies and personalized nutritional strategies in clinical practice, with implications for improving patient outcomes and public health policies.

Keywords: VASER liposuction, ketogenic diet, obesity management, body contouring, BMI above 35, skin retraction, multidisciplinary approach, metabolic health

1. Introduction

Obesity remains one of the most pressing public health concerns globally, contributing significantly to metabolic disorders, cardiovascular diseases, and reduced quality of life. According to the World Health Organization (WHO), the prevalence of obesity has more than tripled since 1975, with over 650 million adults now classified as obese. This growing epidemic is influenced by a complex interplay of socioeconomic, cultural, and environmental factors, including urbanization, sedentary lifestyles, and the widespread availability of energy-dense foods.

Cultural attitudes toward body image and dietary habits also play a pivotal role in the global rise of obesity. In many regions, high-calorie diets rich in refined sugars and fats have become normalized, while physical activity levels have decreased due to technological advancements and urban infrastructure favoring automobile use over active transportation. These trends exacerbate health disparities, as economically disadvantaged populations often have limited access to nutritious foods and safe spaces for exercise.

The consequences of obesity extend beyond physical health, impacting mental well-being, social inclusion, and healthcare systems worldwide. Traditional weight loss interventions, such as caloric restriction and exercise, frequently fall short for individuals with a BMI above 35, necessitating innovative solutions. While bariatric surgery offers significant weight loss potential, it is often accompanied by risks, high costs, and extensive recovery periods.

Recent advancements in medical and esthetic technologies have provided alternative pathways for addressing obesity. VASER liposuction, a sophisticated ultrasound-assisted technique, has emerged as a minimally invasive option capable of reducing fat deposits while enhancing skin tightening through collagen remodeling [1]. Simultaneously, the ketogenic diet, a high-fat, low-carbohydrate nutritional strategy, promotes sustained fat loss and metabolic regulation by inducing a state of ketosis. Together, these approaches offer a dual solution, addressing both the esthetic and metabolic challenges associated with obesity.

This chapter explores the integration of VASER liposuction and the ketogenic diet as a holistic strategy for obesity management. By analyzing clinical outcomes, patient satisfaction, and long-term benefits, we aim to demonstrate the transformative potential of this combined approach, emphasizing its role in bridging the gap between traditional weight loss methods and bariatric surgery. According to the World Health Organization (WHO), more than 650 million adults worldwide suffer from obesity, with numbers continuing to increase at an alarming rate. Conventional weight loss strategies, including caloric restriction, physical activity, and pharmacotherapy, often prove insufficient for individuals with a BMI above 35. While bariatric surgery remains a primary option for severe obesity, it carries inherent risks, prolonged recovery, and long-term complications.

Recent advancements in esthetic surgery and metabolic health management have led to a growing interest in minimally invasive alternatives for body contouring and weight reduction. Specifically, technological innovations in VASER liposuction have addressed significant limitations of traditional methods [2]. Unlike conventional suction-assisted liposuction, VASER employs ultrasound-assisted technology to emulsify fat selectively, preserving vital structures such as nerves and connective tissues. This precision minimizes postoperative irregularities and enhances skin tightening by stimulating collagen production, a critical factor for high BMI patients prone to skin laxity. Furthermore, the ketogenic diet complements these esthetic advancements by leveraging metabolic science to optimize fat oxidation and improve hormonal balance. Together, these methods provide a comprehensive solution for patients seeking both immediate and sustained results. VASER liposuction, a refined ultrasound-assisted technique, has gained prominence due to its ability to selectively target adipose tissue while preserving vital structures such as blood vessels and connective tissues. Unlike traditional suction-assisted liposuction (SAL), VASER liposuction enhances skin contraction and collagen remodeling, making it a valuable tool in patients with high BMI who are prone to skin laxity post-weight loss.

Simultaneously, the ketogenic diet has emerged as a powerful nutritional strategy for sustainable fat loss and metabolic regulation. By inducing a state of ketosis, where the body shifts from glucose to fat oxidation as its primary energy source, the ketogenic diet promotes weight loss, improves insulin sensitivity, and reduces systemic inflammation. Research by Schreiber et al. [3] highlights the hormonal changes post-liposuction that enhance metabolic benefits, while studies by Chia et al. [4] emphasize the precision and efficacy of VASER liposuction in achieving both esthetic and metabolic outcomes.

Furthermore, De La Cruz et al. [5] underline the role of lipoplasty in regulating metabolic profiles, showcasing its potential to complement dietary interventions for holistic patient management. These findings align with emerging clinical evidence, reinforcing the combined utility of VASER liposuction and the ketogenic diet in achieving optimal outcomes.

This chapter presents a comprehensive analysis of the combined effects of VASER liposuction and a ketogenic diet in a cohort of high BMI patients. These findings offer valuable insights into how advanced medical technologies and personalized nutritional strategies can address the multifaceted challenges of obesity. By focusing on both esthetic and metabolic outcomes, this approach underscores the potential for innovative, minimally invasive techniques to bridge existing gaps in obesity management. By examining clinical outcomes, metabolic improvements, and patient satisfaction, we aim to highlight the potential of this approach as a viable alternative to conventional weight loss interventions and bariatric surgery.

2. Methods

2.1 Patient selection

A retrospective case series analysis was conducted on 10 high BMI patients (>35) who underwent VASER liposuction followed by a structured ketogenic diet. The case series includes patients representing a diverse range of cultural and ethnic backgrounds, providing valuable insights into the adaptability of the combined approach across different populations. Patients ranged in age from 23 to 53 years, with a balanced representation of genders, highlighting the broad appeal and applicability of this intervention. The inclusion criteria required patients to be in good general health, non-smokers, and committed to following a ketogenic diet postoperatively. Patients with severe systemic illnesses, uncontrolled diabetes, or contraindications to surgery were excluded.

2.2 Surgical procedure

VASER liposuction was performed under sedation or general anesthesia, depending on the extent of fat removal and patient preference. All procedures were conducted as day-care surgeries, allowing patients to be discharged on the same day. Target areas for fat aspiration varied based on gender:

- *Men:* Abdomen, flanks, back, and chest.
- *Women:* Abdomen, flanks, back, arms, thighs, knees, and calves.

A tumescent solution containing saline, lidocaine, bicarbonate, and epinephrine was infiltrated into the target areas to minimize bleeding, reduce pain, and facilitate fat emulsification. Following this, a VASER probe with either a 3.7 two-ring or three-ring tip was employed to selectively break down adipose tissue while preserving connective tissues, blood vessels, and nerves. The emulsified fat was aspirated using a 3.7 or 4.6 mm cannula, ensuring even fat removal and achieving smooth contours.

Postoperatively, patients were immediately fitted with compression garments to minimize swelling and mitigate potential complications such as seroma formation, asymmetry, or skin irregularities. In some cases, compression boards were used for the abdomen and other areas to provide additional support and improve outcomes. To reduce the risk of bleeding, all patients received transaminic acid injections during the procedure. Antibiotics and oral analgesics were prescribed for at-home recovery.

Postoperative care included:

- Wearing compression garments for 6 weeks.
- Starting lymphatic drainage massages after the first postoperative week, continuing for a month.
- Encouraging early ambulation to prevent complications like deep vein thrombosis (DVT).

This meticulous approach to patient management underscores the importance of combining procedural precision with effective postoperative protocols to ensure optimal outcomes. *The introduction of a structured ketogenic diet post-surgery further enhanced the results,* promoting sustained weight loss, improved metabolic health, and high patient satisfaction.

2.3 Ketogenic diet protocol

A structured ketogenic diet, initiated 5 days post-surgery, included high-protein and healthy fats. This 6-month regimen was monitored by a dietitian, focusing on metabolic parameters and weight reduction.

3. Results

3.1 Patient demographics

3.1.1 Clinical outcomes

- *Weight loss percentages:* Patients exhibited an average weight loss of 5–12% over 6–12 months.
- *BMI improvements:* Mean BMI reduction ranged from three to nine points postoperatively.

- *Esthetic outcomes:* All patients demonstrated enhanced body contouring and improved skin tightening, as confirmed through clinical evaluation and photographic documentation.

- *Metabolic improvements:* Sevety per cent of patients reported improved glycemic control, reduced triglyceride levels, or better insulin sensitivity.

- *Patient satisfaction:* Average satisfaction score was 9/10, reflecting positive experiences with both the procedure and postoperative results.

3.2 Representative cases

Case 1: A 36-year-old male with a BMI of 40.9 underwent VASER liposuction targeting the abdomen, flanks, and chest. Postoperative BMI was reduced to 31.0, and it was accompanied by improved energy levels and reduced triglyceride levels.

Case 2: A 25-year-old female with a BMI of 37 underwent upper and lower-body contouring with VASER liposuction and adhered strictly to the ketogenic diet. She experienced a weight reduction of 32 kg over 12 months, achieving a BMI of 22.6 and significant improvement in PCOS symptoms.

Case 3: A 41-year-old female with a BMI of 35 underwent multiple VASER liposuction procedures and achieved a weight loss of 35 kg over 12 months, with no significant skin laxity or complications.

Case 4: A 53-year-old male with a BMI of 35 underwent VASER liposuction targeting the abdomen and chest. He demonstrated improved glycemic control and sustained visceral fat reduction at 6 months postoperatively.

3.3 Summary of trends and insights

3.3.1 Gender-specific improvements

- *Men:* Reductions in triglyceride levels and improved hypertension management.

- *Women:* Improved insulin sensitivity, symptom alleviation from polycystic ovary syndrome (PCOS), and better weight maintenance.

- *Complication rates:* Minimal bruising and transient swelling were noted but resolved without intervention.

- *Sustainability:* Patients adhering to the ketogenic diet showed better maintenance of weight loss and metabolic benefits compared to those who deviated (**Table 1**).

Table 2 displays improvements in triglyceride levels, blood sugar, and blood pressure.

- *Immediate outcomes:* VASER liposuction achieved significant fat reduction, with an average midsection circumference decrease of 8–15 cm.

- *Long-term outcomes:* Over 6–12 months, adherence to the ketogenic diet led to additional weight loss (5–12% of body weight), visceral fat reduction, and improved skin tightening.

Patient satisfaction exceeded 90%, and minimal complications were reported.

SN	Age (years)	Gender	Procedure	Presurgery weight (kg)	Presurgery BMI	After Surgery Weight (kg)	After surgery BMI	Complications (if any)	Patient satisfaction (1–10)
1	24	Female	VASER liposuction Multiple areas	91.3	35	76	26.6	None	9
2	53	Male	VASER Liposuction chest, Abdomen and flanks	100.8	35	96	32	Minimal bruising	8
3	35	Male	VASER liposuction of thighs and buttocks	109.7	36.6	105.9	35.3	Swelling	7
4	37	Male	VASER liposuction of abdomen, flanks, back, and chest	113.9	35	93	28	None	9
5	25	Female	VASER liposuction of full abdomen and arms	83.3	37	51	22.6	None	10
6	40	Male	VASER Liposuciton of Abdomen and chest	118	36.1	101	31.1	Minimal discomfort	9
7	36	Male	VASER liposuction of chest, abdomen, and flanks	127	40.9	97	31	None	10
8	23	Female	VASER liposuction of abdomen & Flanks	91	37	61	23	None	10
9	36	Female	VASER liposuction of thighs and calves	109	39	65	23	Swelling	8
10	41	Female	Multiple VASER liposuction procedures	90	35	55	21	None	10

Table 1.
Patient characteristics, procedural details, and outcomes following VASER liposuction and ketogenic diet in individuals with BMI above 35: a summary of pre- and post-surgery weight and BMI, complications, and patient satisfaction scores.

Parameter	Preintervention	Postintervention
Triglycerides (mg/dL)	Increased in four patients	Normalized in three patients
Blood sugar levels	High in three patients	Improved levels in all patients
Blood pressure	Elevated in two patients	Improved in both patients

Table 2.
Metabolic changes postintervention.

4. Discussion

Drawing from my clinical experience, VASER liposuction has shown remarkable results in high BMI patients by significantly reducing fat volume while improving skin elasticity. However, despite its advantages, there are limitations and challenges associated with its application in high BMI patients. One of the primary concerns is its suitability for extreme obesity cases. While VASER liposuction is effective in body contouring, it is not a weight loss solution on par with bariatric surgery. Patients with extremely high BMIs may require multiple sessions to achieve satisfactory results, and the amount of fat that can be safely removed in a single procedure is limited due to safety guidelines.

Another important factor to consider is the cost implications. Compared to traditional liposuction techniques, VASER liposuction tends to be more expensive due to the advanced technology and specialized training required for its use. This may limit its accessibility to patients from lower socioeconomic backgrounds, making it a less viable option for widespread obesity management.

Additionally, postoperative care is crucial for ensuring optimal results. Compression garments, lymphatic drainage massages, and strict adherence to dietary modifications, such as the ketogenic diet, are necessary for maintaining long-term benefits. Patients who do not comply with these recommendations may experience suboptimal outcomes or weight regain over time.

Despite these challenges, VASER liposuction remains a valuable tool for individuals seeking a minimally invasive alternative to bariatric surgery. The combination of body contouring and metabolic benefits through the ketogenic diet presents a promising approach for sustainable weight management and improved quality of life. Among my treated patients, those with a BMI above 35 demonstrated substantial improvements in their metabolic health postoperatively, particularly when adhering to a ketogenic diet. Many of my male patients reported reductions in triglyceride levels and improved hypertension control, while female patients exhibited enhanced insulin sensitivity and better PCOS symptom management [5].

The integration of advanced ultrasound-assisted liposuction, as highlighted by Chia et al. [4], underscores the precision and efficacy of VASER in achieving skin tightening and improved body contour. Compared to traditional liposuction techniques, such as suction-assisted liposuction (SAL) and power-assisted liposuction (PAL), VASER employs ultrasound waves to selectively emulsify fat while preserving blood vessels, nerves, and connective tissue [6]. This results in reduced postoperative bruising and swelling, as well as enhanced collagen remodeling, leading to improved skin contraction.

Emerging technologies such as laser-assisted liposuction (LAL) and radiofrequency-assisted liposuction (RFAL) have also gained traction in body contouring. While LAL utilizes thermal energy to disrupt fat cells, its efficacy in skin tightening is often limited compared to VASER. RFAL, on the other hand, delivers radiofrequency energy to induce skin contraction, but studies suggest that VASER achieves more uniform fat removal with less risk of burns or thermal damage. Additionally, VASER's ability to target dense, fibrous fat makes it particularly advantageous for male chest contouring and secondary liposuction procedures where scar tissue may be present. By leveraging its advanced emulsification capabilities, VASER remains a leading choice in modern body contouring procedures. Moreover, De La Cruz et al. [5] reported that lipoplasty not only aids in esthetic outcomes but also contributes to metabolic regulation, a finding mirrored in this study's cohort.

This approach synergizes esthetic and metabolic benefits. VASER liposuction contributes to skin tightening through ultrasound-assisted technology that promotes collagen remodeling. This enhances skin elasticity and provides a more contoured appearance, as observed in **Figures 1B** and **2B** [7]. Concurrently, the ketogenic diet aids in metabolic health by inducing ketosis, a state where the body utilizes stored fat as a primary energy source, thereby reducing visceral fat and improving lipid profiles [8].

VASER-assisted lipoplasty (VAL) demonstrates remarkable benefits in body contouring, including superior skin tightening and reduced blood loss compared to traditional suction-assisted lipoplasty (SAL). A multicenter, prospective, randomized trial highlights a statistically significant 53% improvement in skin retraction with VAL, attributed to its ultrasound-assisted technology that stimulates collagen remodeling. Furthermore, the study found a 26% reduction in blood loss with VAL compared to SAL, underscoring its safety profile during high-volume fat removal procedures [9].

These findings align with the outcomes observed in our case series. Patients reported significant esthetic improvements, particularly in skin tightening, without the need for additional procedures to address skin laxity. The capacity of VAL to preserve vital structures while emulsifying fat enhances the precision of fat removal, which is especially critical for high BMI patients prone to uneven contouring and skin sagging post-weight loss.

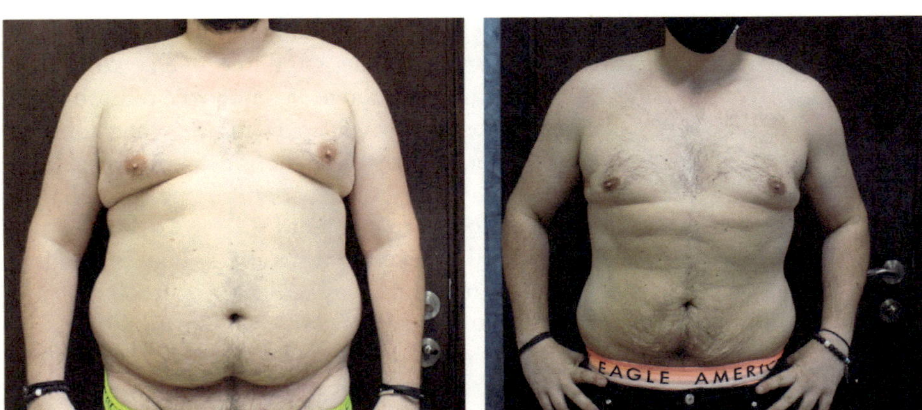

(A) (B)

Figure 1.
(A) Front preoperative views of chest, abdomen, and flanks in a high BMI male patient (see Section 3.2).
(B) Six-month postoperative results showcasing significant fat reduction and skin tightening (see Section 3.2).

DOI: http://dx.doi.org/10.5772/intechopen.1009622

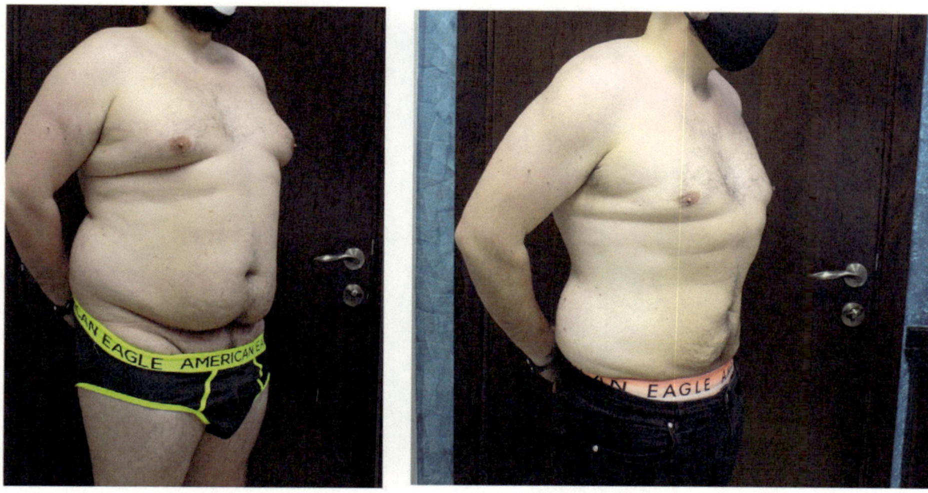

(A) (B)

Figure 2.
(A) Side preoperative views of chest, abdomen, and flanks in a high BMI male patient (see Section 3.2).
(B) Six-month side view postoperative results showing significant skin retraction (see Section 3.2).

Additionally, VAL's capability to minimize blood loss facilitates smoother post-operative recovery, which was evident in our cohort, where complication rates were minimal and recovery times were expedited. This further supports VAL as a preferred choice for body contouring in both high and low BMI patients, offering consistent esthetic and metabolic benefits.

In male patients, reductions in triglyceride levels and hypertension management were significant, correlating with better cardiovascular outcomes (**Figure 3D**) [10]. Female patients benefited from improved insulin sensitivity, relief from PCOS symptoms, and sustainable weight maintenance, as highlighted in **Figure 4B**. Schreiber et al. [3] noted that hormonal changes post-liposuction, including adjustments in ghrelin and adiponectin levels, further enhance the metabolic benefits when combined with dietary modifications.

These outcomes emphasize the dual efficacy of this integrated approach for achieving esthetic and metabolic improvements, providing a viable alternative to traditional bariatric procedures for select high BMI patients.

Long-term follow-up of patients revealed that those who adhered to the ketogenic diet maintained their weight loss and metabolic improvements, whereas non-adherent patients exhibited weight regain [11]. These findings reinforce the need for integrated dietary interventions post-liposuction to sustain long-term benefits [12, 13].

Even without the incorporation of the ketogenic diet, VASER liposuction alone has demonstrated significant weight loss and BMI reduction in patients. A study by Kandulu et al. [14] analyzed 51 patients undergoing VASER-assisted liposuction and observed a substantial decrease in body weight and BMI within a month of the procedure. Interestingly, the study highlighted that factors such as gender, age, aspiration volume, and fat volume had no direct correlation with the weight reduction achieved, suggesting the inherent efficacy of the VASER technology itself. This aligns with my clinical experience, where patients, irrespective of dietary adherence, reported weight loss following the procedure (**Figure 5**).

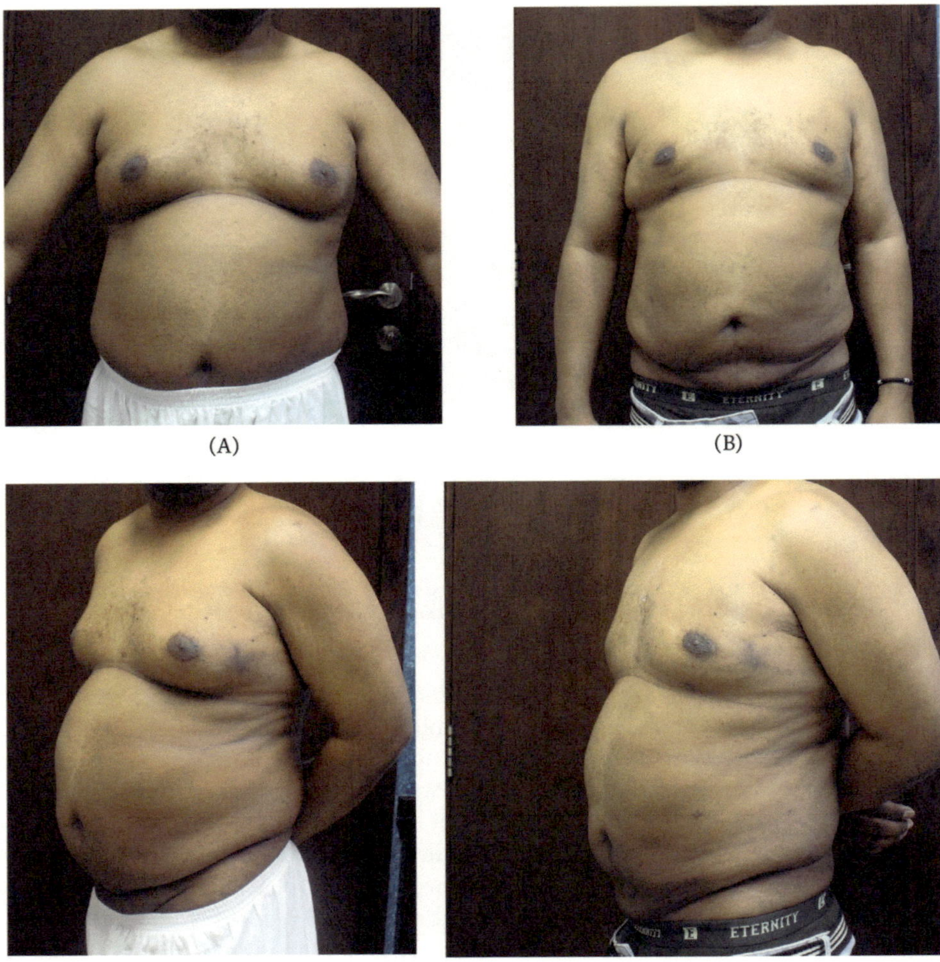

(A) (B) (C) (D)

Figure 3.
(A) and (C) Preoperative front and lateral views of a male patient undergoing VASER liposuction of the chest, abdomen, and flanks (see Section 3.2). (B) and (D) Three-month postoperative front and lateral views illustrating moderate weight loss and improved contour (see Section 3.2).

The findings reinforce the concept that the precision and efficiency of VASER liposuction not only contribute to esthetic outcomes but also have a measurable impact on physical metrics such as weight and BMI. Patients with higher baseline BMIs often benefit more significantly, experiencing reductions in triglyceride levels and improvements in metabolic parameters. These outcomes underscore VASER liposuction's potential as a standalone tool for targeted weight loss in patients not opting for complementary dietary regimens.

However, the absence of a dietary strategy like the ketogenic diet may limit the metabolic benefits post-liposuction, particularly in addressing systemic issues like insulin resistance or chronic inflammation. Future studies could investigate the comparative outcomes of VASER liposuction alone versus in conjunction with structured dietary programs, further elucidating the comprehensive impact of these methodologies in obesity management (**Figure 6**).

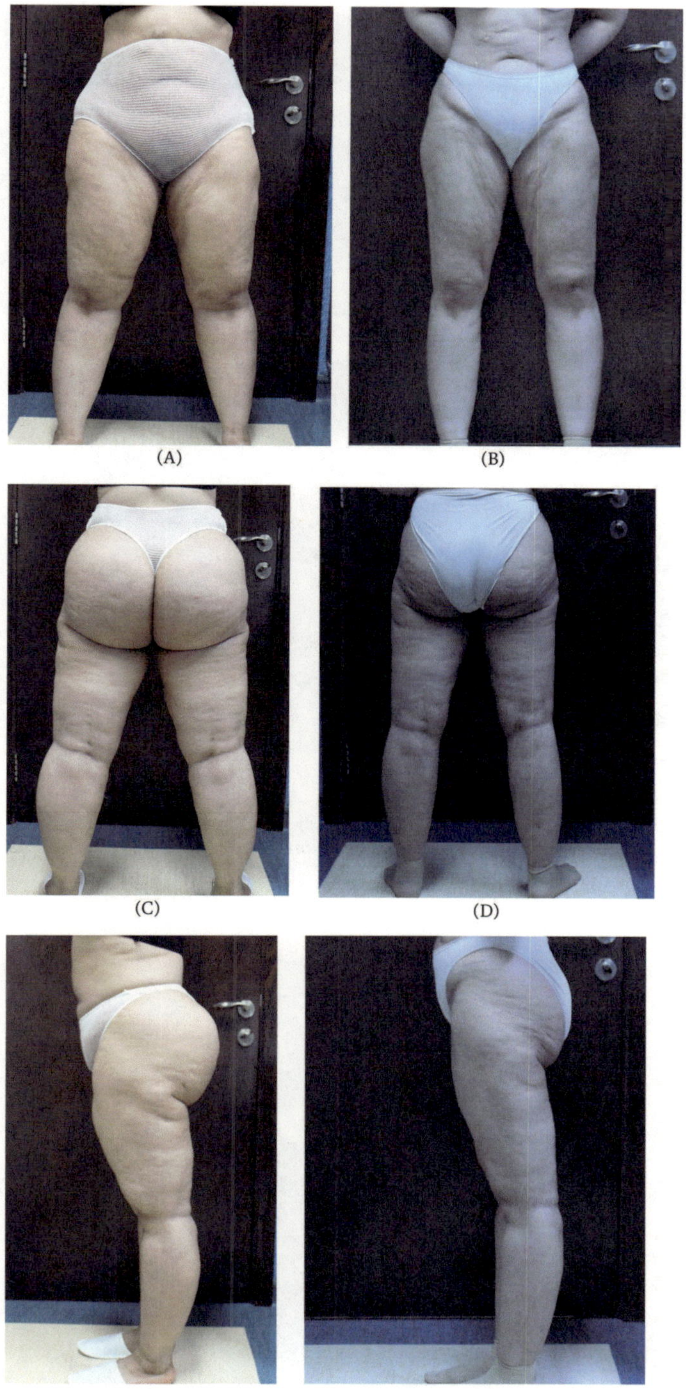

(A) (B) (C) (D) (E) (F)

Figure 4.
(A) Front view of lower limbs (thighs and knees) preoperatively (see Section 3.2). (B) Long-term postoperative results of thighs and knees showing enhanced contour (see Section 3.2). (C) Back view of thighs and calves preoperatively (see Section 3.2). (D) Long-term results (3 years post-op) illustrating sustained improvement (see Section 3.2). (E) Side view of thighs and calves preoperatively (see Section 3.2). (F) Long-term postoperative results showing improved contour and skin quality (see Section 3.2).

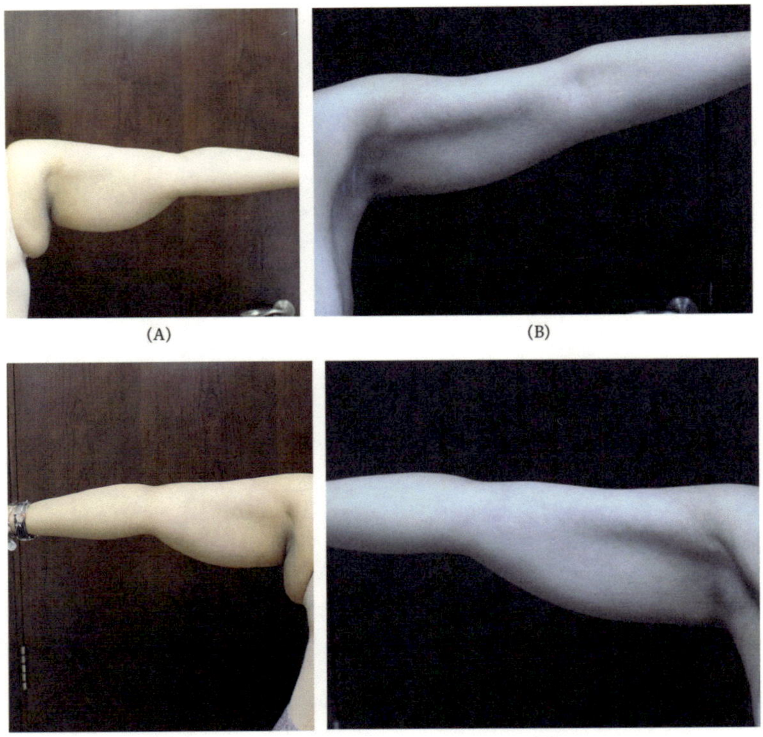

(A) (B) (C) (D)

Figure 5.
(A) and (C) Front views of right and left arms demonstrating fatty deposits and loose skin. (B) and (D) improved contouring and skin tightening sustained results 3 years postoperatively (see Section 3.2).

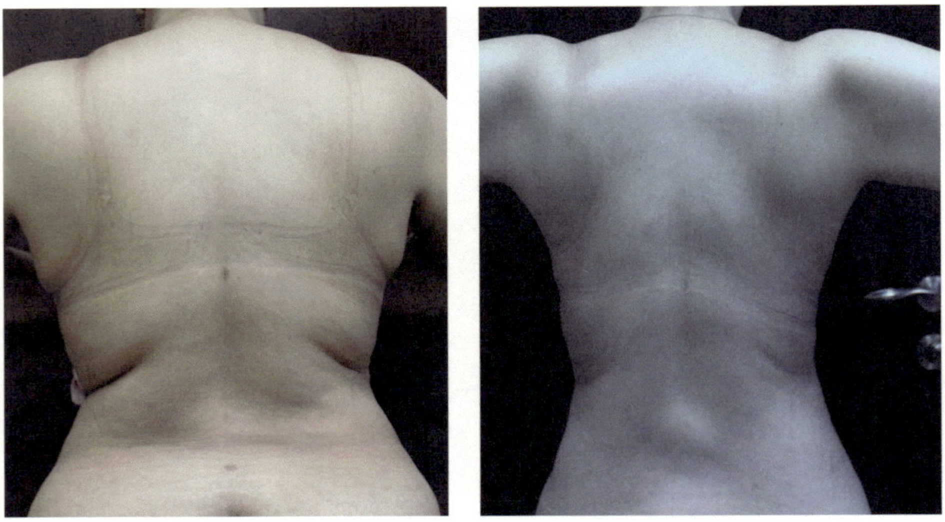

(A) (B)

Figure 6.
(A) and (B) Long-term results of back folds after massive weight loss and VASER liposuction, showing improved skin elasticity and contour (see Section 3.2).

5. Side effects and challenges

5.1 Common postoperative complications

- *Skin laxity:* Some patients experienced skin laxity post-weight loss especially those who regained weight or after pregnancy in female phenotype [15].
- *Contour irregularities:* Noted in patients who did not adhere to dietary recommendations, leading to uneven fat redistribution.
- *Swelling and bruising:* Common postoperative effects, all of which resolved within weeks.
- *Limited metabolic improvement:* Patients with normal preoperative metabolic markers did not experience significant changes in lipid or glucose levels.

5.2 Importance of postoperative dietary adherence

- Weight regain was noted in some patients who did not adhere to dietary recommendations, causing fat redistribution and contour irregularities.
- Long-term dietary adherence plays a key role in sustaining both metabolic and esthetic benefits.

5.3 Considerations for best outcomes

5.3.1 Patient selection and preoperative counseling

- Proper *preoperative assessment* is crucial to identify ideal candidates for the combined approach.
- Patients must be counseled on *realistic expectations* and the importance of *postoperative care*.

5.3.2 Role of multidisciplinary follow-up

- A multidisciplinary approach, including *plastic surgeons, nutritionists, and physiotherapists*, enhances long-term success.
- Regular follow-up ensures *early identification of complications and better weight maintenance strategies*.

6. Conclusion

The combination of VASER liposuction and the ketogenic diet represents an innovative, minimally invasive approach to obesity management, particularly for high BMI patients. This synergistic strategy not only delivers remarkable body contouring outcomes but also fosters significant metabolic improvements. VASER liposuction, with its advanced ultrasound-assisted technology, provides enhanced precision, superior skin tightening, and reduced blood loss compared to traditional lipoplasty methods. This makes it a highly effective solution for addressing esthetic challenges, especially in patients prone to skin laxity.

Furthermore, the ketogenic diet complements the procedural outcomes by optimizing fat oxidation, improving glycemic control, and reducing systemic inflammation. Together, these methods have demonstrated the potential to improve overall health, as evidenced by reductions in BMI, enhanced hormonal regulation, and improved cardiovascular metrics observed in our case series.

Notably, even without dietary interventions, VASER liposuction alone has been shown to yield significant weight loss and esthetic benefits, underscoring its standalone efficacy. However, integrating a structured ketogenic regimen amplifies these effects, enabling sustained weight management and metabolic stability.

Future research should aim to expand follow-up periods, refine patient selection criteria, and explore additional adjunct therapies to further enhance outcomes. This chapter underscores the transformative potential of combining advanced surgical techniques with personalized nutritional strategies, offering a viable alternative to bariatric surgery and bridging the gap in obesity management for diverse patient populations.

Funding acknowledgments

No funding was obtained for this study.

Ethical approvals

This study was approved by the institutional review board.

Future research directions

Future studies should focus on randomized controlled trials to validate the observed outcomes. Extended follow-up periods are essential to assess the long-term sustainability of weight loss and metabolic improvements. Additionally, exploring the molecular mechanisms underlying collagen remodeling in VASER liposuction and the systemic anti-inflammatory effects of the ketogenic diet could further substantiate this combined approach.

Author details

Hasan Ali
Medical Director and Plastic Surgeon, Hasan Surgery FZ LLC, Dubai Healthcare City, Dubai, UAE

*Address all correspondence to: hasan@hasansurgery.com

References

[1] Ruff PG et al. Consensus-based recommendations for ultrasound-assisted liposuction. Plastic and Reconstructive Surgery. Global Open. 2023;**11**(7):e5110. DOI: 10.1097/GOX.0000000000005110

[2] Gingrass MK, Kenkel JM. Comparing ultrasound-assisted lipoplasty with suction-assisted lipoplasty. Clinics in Plastic Surgery. 1999;**26**(2):283-2ix

[3] Schreiber JE, Singh NK, Shermak MA. The effect of liposuction and diet on ghrelin, adiponectin, and leptin levels in obese Zucker rats. Plastic and Reconstructive Surgery. 2006;**117**(6):1829-1835

[4] Chia CT, Neinstein RM, Theodorou SJ. Evidence-based medicine: Liposuction. Plastic and Reconstructive Surgery. 2017;**139**(1):267e-274e. DOI: 10.1097/PRS.0000000000002859

[5] De La Cruz E. Lipoplasty in the overweight patient. Clinics in Plastic Surgery. 2024;**51**(1):29-43. DOI: 10.1016/j.cps.2023.06.010

[6] de Souza Pinto EB, Abdala PC, Maciel CM, dos Santos FP, de Souza RP. Liposuction and VASER. Clinics in Plastic Surgery. 2006;**33**(1):107-vii. DOI: 10.1016/j.cps.2005.09.001

[7] Ali H. Successful outcome of VASER liposuction followed by Keto diet in a 35-year-old man with class III obesity. Plastic and Reconstructive Surgery. Global Open. 2024;**12**(8):e6098

[8] Baylie T, Ayelgn T, Tiruneh M, Tesfa KH. Effect of ketogenic diet on obesity and other metabolic disorders: Narrative review. Diabetes, Metabolic Syndrome and Obesity. 2024;**17**:1391-1401. DOI: 10.2147/DMSO.S447659

[9] Nagy MW, Vanek PF Jr. A multicenter, prospective, randomized, single-blind, controlled clinical trial comparing VASER-assisted Lipoplasty and suction-assisted Lipoplasty. Plastic and Reconstructive Surgery. 2012;**129**(4):681e-689e. DOI: 10.1097/PRS.0b013e3182442274

[10] Lanzano G, Napoli F, et al. Correlation between BMI, fat aspirate volume, and complications in VASER liposuction. JPRAS Open. 2024;**42**:170-177. DOI: 10.1016/j.jpra.2024.08.007

[11] Davis W, Lawrence N. Weight loss: How does it fit in with liposuction? Dermatologic Surgery. 2020;**46** (Suppl. 1):S22-S28. DOI: 10.1097/DSS.0000000000002225

[12] Esposito K, Giugliano G, Giugliano D. Metabolic effects of liposuction--yes or no? The New England Journal of Medicine. 2004;**351**(13):1354-1357. DOI: 10.1056/NEJM200409233511320

[13] González-Ortiz M, Robles-Cervantes JA, Cárdenas-Camarena L, Bustos-Saldaña R, Martínez-Abundis E. The effects of surgically removing subcutaneous fat on the metabolic profile and insulin sensitivity in obese women after large-volume liposuction treatment. Hormone and Metabolic Research. 2002;**34**(8):446-449. DOI: 10.1055/s-2002-33603

[14] Kandulu H. Weight loss after VASER-assisted liposuction. Aesthetic Plastic Surgery. 2024;**48**(6):1166-1173. DOI: 10.1007/s00266-023-03775-4

[15] Swanson E. Improved skin contraction after VASER-assisted lipoplasty: Is it a change we can believe in? Plastic and Reconstructive Surgery. 2012;**130**(5):754e-756e. DOI: 10.1097/PRS.0b013e318267d96a